AGELESS FITNESS

At 40 and Beyond

Pankaj Patil

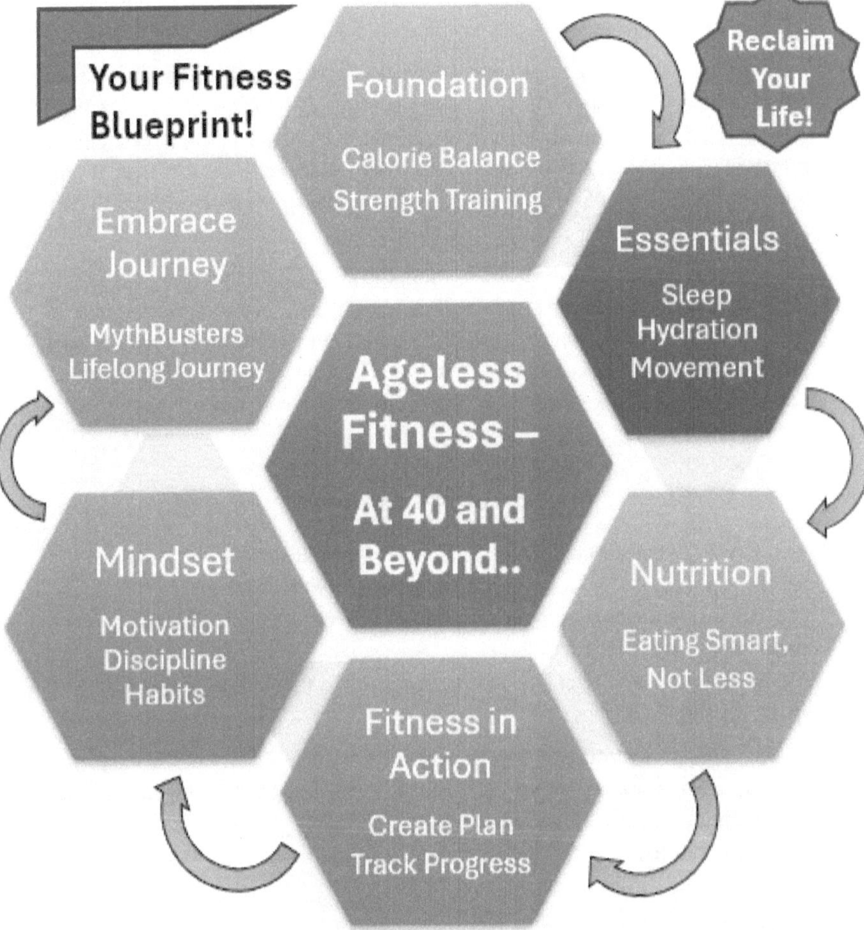

Unlocking Your Best Version At Any Age...

Also included: a companion website - your ultimate hub for tools, templates, and resources to supercharge your fitness journey!

Ageless Fitness - At 40 and Beyond

Turning 40 doesn't mean slowing down - it's the perfect time to take control of your health, build strength, and feel your best. *Ageless Fitness - At 40 and Beyond* is more than just a book; it's a **blueprint for your fitness journey,** equipping you with the knowledge and tools to **become your own fitness guide.**

Covering everything from **calorie balance and strength training to sleep, hydration, movement, and supplements,** this book **simplifies fitness science** into practical, easy-to-follow steps. You'll learn how to **design a personalized plan, track progress effectively, debunk common myths, and make sustainable choices** that fit into your lifestyle, track progress without stress, and develop the **right mindset to stay motivated.**

Although designed for those **40 and beyond,** the principles in this book apply at any age—whether you're starting fresh at 30, 50, or beyond, the fundamentals remain the same. Plus, a **companion website** offers **workout guides, meal planners, and additional resources** to keep you on track. *Ageless Fitness* helps you break barriers and redefine what's possible at any age. **Your fittest years are still ahead—let's get started!**

About the Author

Pankaj Patil is a **Consulting Leader** at a global IT firm and an **INFS-certified nutrition and fitness coach.** After years of putting **wellness on the backburner,** he realized that **staying fit after 40** required a different approach - one that was **practical, sustainable, and backed by science.** Determined to bridge the gap between **fitness myths and real-world solutions,** he set out to share his insights with others facing the same struggles.

Ageless Fitness – At 40 and Beyond was born from this mission. Drawing from both **personal experience and professional expertise,** Pankaj simplifies **fitness into actionable steps** that busy individuals can realistically follow. His focus is on **long-term results,** proving that no matter your **age or starting point, your best fitness years are still ahead.**

Pankaj is an **avid traveller** who enjoys exploring both **Indian and global destinations.** For him, travel is not just about visiting new places but also about **immersing himself in the local culture.** He believes that **food is an integral part of a region's identity** and loves experiencing **local cuisines** wherever he goes. His passion for **travel and food** aligns with his philosophy of living a **balanced, fulfilling life** - one that embraces both **health and enjoyment.**

Through this book, he hopes to **challenge outdated notions** about **aging and fitness,** showing that **strength, health, and vitality** are within reach at **any stage of life.**

CONTENTS

Introduction

Chapter 1: Why 40 is the New 30 34

Part 1
The Foundation

Chapter 2: The Golden Rule – Calorie Balance 42

Contents

Part 3
Nutrition - Eating Smart, Not Less

Contents

ACKNOWLEDGEMENTS

Here we are, at the end of what feels like both a marathon and a sprint, all rolled into one. As I reach the conclusion of this book, I'm overwhelmed with gratitude. This journey has been a mix of determination, self-discovery, and the quiet strength that comes from knowing you're not alone. Every step - through the challenges and the triumphs - has been made easier by the incredible people who stood by me, cheered me on, and believed in this vision. I couldn't have done it without them, and this is my chance to say thank you

First and foremost, I am deeply grateful to **Rishi Darda, Jitendra Chouksey (JC), and Sonali Kulkarni** for their unwavering belief in this book. I am honored to have their golden words grace these pages, offering wisdom and insights that will inspire readers.

Rishi Darda, Joint Managing Director and Editorial Director of Lokmat Media Group, thank you for lending your voice to this book through a thoughtful and motivating foreword. Your generosity, guidance, and faith in this mission have been instrumental in this journey. Your contribution has made this endeavor even more meaningful, and I truly appreciate your trust and encouragement.

JC (Jitendra Chouksey) - the visionary CEO behind Fittr. Your leadership has transformed countless lives, mine included. You've been a guiding force, helping me build not just a stronger body but also a resilient mindset. Without Fittr, I might never have found my path to fitness, and this book wouldn't exist today! Thank you, JC - you've inspired millions, and your impact on the community is immeasurable.

A heartfelt thanks to the amazing **Sonali Kulkarni** for contributing a deeply personal and inspiring note to this book. As an acclaimed actor and writer, your passion extends far beyond the arts—it also encompasses health and well-being. Your friendship with Sonal has been an incredible source of strength, and your fitness journey continues to inspire those around you. You not only light up and bring alive the silver screen but also touch and brighten so many lives with your warmth and authenticity. Thank you for standing with us and supporting this mission of transformation with your remarkable spirit.

To my incredible wife, **Sonal** - you're not just my better half; you're my workout partner, my nutrition expert, and the one who keeps me accountable. Your energy is contagious, and your encouragement has been my secret weapon throughout this process. Thank you for keeping my macros in check and for reminding me that rest days matter just as much as workout days. This book wouldn't have been possible without your constant motivation and push.

Vihaan, my 18-year-old son, a whirlwind of energy who keeps me on my toes. Whether it's devouring every snack in the house or challenging me to stay updated with the latest tech trends, you've been a constant source of inspiration. The way you've taken charge of your fitness at such a young age is truly admirable - keep it up, buddy!

Vera, my four-legged fitness partner - you deserve a medal for all the walks, runs, and those playful moments when I was deep in writing. You remind me daily that fitness is as much about joy and companionship as it is about reps and sets.

To my incredible **Fittr coaches - Manvit Kaur, Vijay Tambi, Sandeep Rawat,** and **Tanya Vahi** - you've been my compass, guiding me, challenging me, and, let's be honest, keeping me sane. Your expertise and tough love have been game-changers.

A special mention to **Manvit**, who is truly one of a kind. Mine and Sonal's journey began with her - our rock-solid mentor, trusted guide, and constant source of inspiration. She has played a pivotal role in shaping our path with her knowledge, dedication, and boundless support. Even today, she remains our **Chief Inspiration Officer**, a title she wears effortlessly. Words cannot fully capture our gratitude for her profound impact on our lives.

A big nod to my dear friend **Yogita Patil**, who started me on this adventure. You nudged (or maybe pushed!) Sonal and me into the Fittr community, and it made all the difference.

A big thank you to **Nilesh Lohia** - more than just a friend, you've been a constant pillar of support through every phase of my journey. From meaningful conversations to those moments of unspoken understanding, your presence has always made a difference. I truly appreciate your friendship and the forever encouragement you've given me along the way!

A huge thank you to **Santosh Mhatre**, way beyond a friend - a rock-solid force and a true companion who's been by my side since the days when life was all about dreams, ambitions, and endless possibilities. From then to now, through every phase, your friendship has been a constant - one that needs no words, just a knowing nod. Grateful for all the shared memories and the ones still to come!

To my **Mother**, whose love and wisdom continue to guide me even in her absence. Your values, strength, and belief in me have been the foundation of everything I've accomplished. This book is as much a tribute to you as it is a reflection of my journey.

To my **Sister Aparna, brother-in-law Kamlesh,** and **my wonderful niece** and **nephew, Aditi** and **Aditya** - your support, encouragement, and the joy you bring into my life have been invaluable. Thank you for always being there and for cheering me on.

To my **in-laws** - your warmth and kindness have been a pillar of strength. Thank you for always standing by us and for fostering a home filled with love and care.

To my colleagues and friends at **LTIMindtree** worldwide, thank you for your continuous support. And a special shout-out to the state-of-the-art gym at the Mensa campus - your space allowed me to squeeze in quick workouts between meetings, making this journey a little less stressful and a lot more rewarding!

To **Flex Fitness Gym** - my fortress of strength (literally). Thank you to all the trainers (special thanks to my coach and buddy **Tanmay**) and fellow members for the motivation, the challenges, and the occasional reality check when I aimed a little too high with the weights. You've been my go-to place to push my limits and, sometimes, to remind me that today is not the day for that extra set.

To my **Band of Brothers - Strikers**. You are more than just 3 am friends; you are the constants in my life who have stood by me through everything. The unfiltered conversations, the laughter, the road-trips, the challenges - we've shared it all. Your steadfast support is truly irreplaceable, and I'm beyond grateful to have you in my corner.

And to the entire **Fittr Community** - you are my tribe, my motivation, and a testament to the power of shared goals. Your stories, struggles, and victories have fueled my own journey, and I am proud to be part of this incredible family.

Finally, to you, **Dear Reader** - thank you for picking up this book. Whether you're just starting out or already deep into your fitness journey, I hope these pages inspire you, challenge you, and maybe even make you smile. Here's to your fitness adventure - may it be fulfilling, rewarding, and fun.

With this book reaching your hands, it's a moment to pause and celebrate - not just the words on these pages, but the journey that made them possible. Whether it's with an energizing workout or a well-deserved treat, it's a reminder that life is about balance - pushing boundaries while cherishing the wins along the way. This isn't the end; it's a milestone - one that marks how far we've come and the endless possibilities still ahead.

Thank you for being part of this journey - here's to the road ahead to Ageless Fitness!

FOREWORD 1: RISHI DARDA, JMD - LOKMAT MEDIA

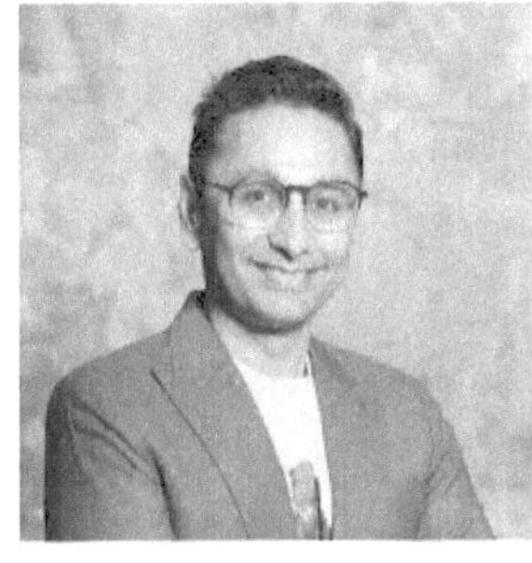

*(Rishi Darda, **Joint Managing Director and Editorial Director of Lokmat Media Group**, is a visionary leader known for his dynamic approach to business and media. With a keen focus on innovation, discipline, and a balanced lifestyle, **his insights inspire countless individuals** to strive for excellence in both personal and professional spheres)*

As I sit down to pen my thoughts, I can't help but reflect on how health and fitness have evolved in my life, especially as I've crossed into my mid-40s. Fitness is no longer about the fleeting moments of vanity or short-term goals - it has become a way of life.

Like many of you, I've battled the whirlwind of balancing work, family, and personal time. But as the years progressed, I realized that investing in my health was no longer optional - it was essential. My 40s brought clarity about the non-negotiables in life, and fitness climbed to the top of that list. Diet discipline became a habit, and structured physical activity became a ritual.

This journey also brought me unexpected joys. About a year ago, I discovered pickleball - a sport I initially dismissed as a passing trend. However, it soon became a passion, thanks to the camaraderie I found on the court. What began as casual games with a group of strangers turned into an enduring bond with a bunch of like-minded individuals. We challenge each other, cheer each other on, and remind one another to keep moving - both on the court and in life. These friendships have added an irreplaceable layer of fun and motivation to my fitness routine.

This book resonates deeply with me because it echoes many of the principles I've come to value. Whether it's the emphasis on strength training, the power of proper hydration, or the crucial role of mindset, this guide offers something for everyone, regardless of where they are on their fitness journey. The chapters on motivation and habits particularly struck a chord, as they are often the unsung heroes of long-term success.

After turning 42, Pankaj was confronted with the harsh reality of how years of neglecting his health had drained his energy, confidence, and ability to enjoy life fully. He embraced the challenges of balancing work, family, and health - took charge of his fitness, and also became a certified nutrition and fitness coach. So I like that his motivation for writing this book comes from his own remarkable transformation.

Fitness after 40 isn't just about reclaiming your body - it's about reclaiming your life. It's about feeling strong, energized, and ready to embrace every opportunity with vigor. I hope this book inspires you as much as my journey continues to inspire me.

Here's to unlocking the best version of yourself - at any age!

Rishi Darda
Jt. Managing Director & Editorial Director, Lokmat Media Group

FOREWORD 2: JC (JITENDRA CHOUKSEY), FOUNDER - FITTR

By JC (Jitendra Chouksey), Founder of Fittr

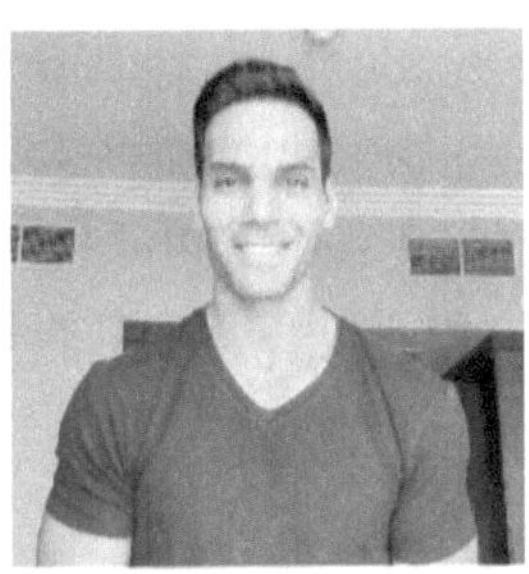

*(Jitendra Chouksey, better known as **JC**, is the driving force behind **Fittr** as its **CEO**. A self-made entrepreneur and the **Businessworld Young Entrepreneur Award** winner, he turned a simple act of helping friends with their fitness goals on WhatsApp into a **thriving global business**. What started as a passion project has now transformed the lives of over **300,000 people worldwide**, created sustainable careers for hundreds, and revolutionized the way fitness is approached. His vision goes beyond just building a business - it's about making health and fitness accessible to everyone, everywhere)*

It's often said that life begins at 40, but for many, this is also the age when health begins to take a backseat. Careers, families, and societal expectations frequently take precedence, leaving little time to prioritize fitness and well-being. However, turning 40 doesn't mean giving up on your health. In fact, it can be the perfect time to embrace a new chapter of vitality and purpose. That's why *Ageless Fitness: At 40 and Beyond* is such a remarkable and much-needed book.

As someone who has dedicated my life to promoting health and fitness, I firmly believe that age is merely a number - it should never be a barrier to achieving a fit, active, and fulfilling lifestyle. This book is a testament to that belief, written by someone who not only understands the challenges of balancing life and fitness firsthand but has overcome them with incredible dedication, discipline, and a commitment to self-improvement.

Pankaj and his wife Sonal have been a part of Fittr family for years. What stands out about Pankaj is his relentless passion for fitness, his unshakable commitment to personal growth, and, above all, his genuine desire to help others. He is not just someone who talks about transformation - he embodies it. His journey is one of resilience, determination, and a refusal to settle for mediocrity.

Pankaj didn't just transform his own life. He became an INFS-certified coach, a mentor, and now an author, dedicated to showing others that turning 40 isn't the beginning of the end - it's the start of something extraordinary. His story is a powerful reminder that it's never too late to redefine your priorities and rewrite your narrative.

What sets this book apart is its deeply practical and relatable approach. Pankaj demystifies the world of fitness for those over 40, proving that it's not about extreme diets, gruelling workouts, or unattainable goals. Instead, he highlights the power of small, sustainable steps - embracing quantified nutrition, incorporating strength training, and making simple yet impactful lifestyle changes. These are the foundations of long-lasting transformations, and the book explains them with clarity, compassion, and a wealth of personal experience.

This book is much more than a fitness guide; it's a roadmap to a healthier, more active, and more fulfilling life. It is packed with actionable insights, personal anecdotes, and motivational guidance that only someone who has lived this journey can provide. Every page reflects the dedication to helping others unlock their true potential, no matter their age or circumstances.

For anyone who has ever wondered if it's too late to start, this book offers an emphatic answer: It's never too late. Whether you're 40, 50, or even 60, you can take charge of your health and unlock a version of yourself you never imagined possible.

I am honoured to write this foreword for this book because it aligns perfectly with Fittr's mission of making fitness accessible and achievable for everyone. Fitness is not just about aesthetics; it's about improving your quality of life, building resilience, and inspiring those around you to do the same.

To everyone holding this book, know that you're in for a transformative experience. Pankaj's story will inspire you; his expertise will empower you, and his practical advice will guide you on every step of your journey.

Here's to embracing ageless fitness and proving that life at 40 - and beyond - can be healthier, stronger, and more vibrant than ever before.

JC
Founder, Fittr
About Fittr

Founded by **Jitendra Chouksey (JC)** in 2014 as a simple WhatsApp group to promote health, **Fittr** has grown into a leading global fitness and nutrition platform. By leveraging cutting-edge technology and expert human coaches, Fittr makes fitness accessible, achievable, and sustainable for all.

With over **300,000 successful transformations** and a thriving community of more than **3 million members**, Fittr offers:

- **Personalized coaching**
- **Customized diet and workout plans**
- **One-on-one personal training**
- **Injury rehabilitation programs**

Driven by its mission to make **50 million people fit** and create meaningful career opportunities in the fitness industry, Fittr continues to inspire, educate, and transform lives worldwide.

For more information, visit www.fittr.com

PERSONAL NOTE: SONALI KULKARNI, ACCOMPLISHED ACTOR AND WRITER

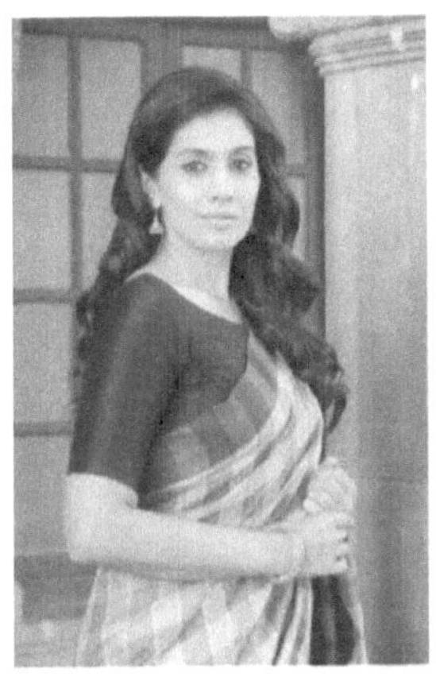

*(Sonali embodies grace, talent, and versatility, making her an endearing and inspirational icon in the **world of cinema**. With her memorable **on-screen performances** and powerful words as a **writer**, she continues to inspire countless individuals by excelling in every role she takes on - both on and off the stage. Her **dedication to fitness and well-being** further highlights her belief in leading a balanced and fulfilling life, making her a role model for many)*

I have known Pankaj and Sonal for more than a decade and a half. Sonal has always been warm and exuberant - her vivacious energy is the first thing that comes to mind when I think of her. She is grounded, focused, and incredibly determined.

I distinctly remember the major shift in her journey - a little before the pandemic. Our conversations and messages had always carried a common thread: fitness.

Fast forward to when I met Pankaj for his upcoming dream project. He looked crisp, fresh, and composed. As he spoke about his book *Ageless Fitness*, I was completely taken by surprise with all the details!

Here is a new fitness dictionary for us!

It captures not just their personal journey but also the challenges they faced along the way. And let's be honest - who doesn't love food? We all do! But Pankaj isn't asking us to stop loving food; instead, he compels us to fall in love with it all over again - only this time, with a deeper understanding. In simple words, he explains the importance of our intake and encourages us to be mindful of the calorie balance.

Once we unlock the fear of this 'math,' the only path ahead is towards becoming fitter. What's even more exciting is that Pankaj has come up with a unique website which provides tools, guidelines and a forum where we can connect with fellow health enthusiasts, learn from their struggles and victories, and fuel our own journey in a positive way.

The beauty of this book lies in its simplicity and practicality. It provides actionable advice on nutrition, exercise, sleep, and overall well-being without overwhelming the reader.

At the end of the day, being healthy is a choice - it's our personal journey. After all, it's literally in our own hands... and our own mouths! ☺

The less we treat it as a burden, in every sense, the richer our lives will be. And honestly, who doesn't like being rich? Cheers, Pankaj! 👍

Warm regards,
Sonali Kulkarni
Actor, Author, and Advocate for Holistic Wellness

THE STORY BEHIND THIS BOOK

It was November 2018, and I had just turned 42 - at the peak of my IT consulting career. My days were filled with back-to-back meetings, urgent client calls, and relentless project deadlines. Evenings? Well, those were usually spent trying to troubleshoot last-minute issues or playing catch-up with the work that never seemed to end. My personal life was just as busy, and time was something I was running short on. Fitness? It was right up there with "learning a new language" and "organizing the study-room" - firmly parked in the "I'll get to it someday" category.

Then one day, I realized "someday" was quietly slipping away. I'd become that guy who struggled to carry grocery bags up the stairs, gasped for air after a short walk or jog, and felt exhausted no matter how much tea or coffee I chugged. My clothes were getting snugger, my energy levels were in free fall, and keeping up with my kid felt like running a marathon with a backpack full of bricks.

There wasn't a dramatic "aha" moment or a sudden health scare - just a slow, creeping realization that if I didn't start taking care of myself, I might not have the chance later. I wanted to be there for my family, keep up with my son, and actually enjoy the life I was working so hard to build.

So, at 42, I decided to make a change. I didn't know much about fitness or nutrition at all, but I knew I had to start somewhere.

I began with small steps-morning walks, running sessions. There were days when I wanted to quit, when the comfort of my couch seemed far more appealing than another run.

However, after 2-3 months of running with no noticeable results, I felt tempted to return to my couch potato ways. Frustration was setting in, and that's when a friend introduced me to the Fittr group (formerly SQUATS), changing our lives forever. My wife, Sonal, and I started this journey together, supported by an our amazing Fittr coach and a motivating community.

We embraced a plan focused on quantified nutrition and strength training, along with improved sleep, hydration, and staying active beyond workouts. Gradually, we began to notice positive changes - we felt stronger, more energetic, and more in control of our health.

The more progress we made, the more curious I became. I immersed myself in books, articles, and research on fitness and nutrition, eager to learn more.

And then I fell in love with the process. What started as a reluctant effort to get healthier turned into a passion for fitness. I wasn't just doing this for myself anymore; I wanted to help others feel the same sense of empowerment and vitality that I had discovered. So, I took the plunge and became a certified nutrition and fitness consultant.

I found a balance I never thought possible - juggling a demanding career with a solid commitment to my health. The best part? I got to help others navigate their own fitness journeys, sharing in their challenges and celebrating their victories.

The core theme of this book is simple yet profound: **fitness after 40 isn't just possible - it's powerful and yes, it is ageless!**

Sure, the body may not bounce back as quickly as it did in your 20s, and recovery might take a little longer, but that doesn't mean you can't achieve impressive results. It's about working smarter, not harder, and understanding that sustainable progress is rooted in realistic goals, consistent habits, and a positive mindset.

But this book isn't just about fitness for those in their 40s and beyond. **There's a chapter dedicated to fitness at any age**, because whether you're 25, 45, or 65, the principles of health and wellness remain largely the same. It's never too late - or too early - to make a positive change. The strategies and techniques shared here are adaptable, ensuring that anyone, regardless of age or fitness level, can benefit from them.

I'm not here to peddle quick fixes or miracle cures. Instead, I want to share the practical strategies, lessons, and tips that worked for me and the people I've guided. I'll show you how to make fitness a sustainable part of your life, no matter how packed your schedule is. And yes, we're going to have some fun and a lot of flexibility along the way - because if there's one thing I've learned, it's that fitness doesn't have to feel like a punishment. It can be an adventure filled with challenges, triumphs, and a good dose of laughs.

If you need extra guidance or just want to chat about your journey, feel free to reach out. I've got a blog full of resources to help you curate your own path, and I'd love to hear how you're doing.

So, let's dive in. Here's to feeling fantastic at 40 and beyond - or whatever age you happen to be!

Stay Fit, Stay Happy, and Discover Ageless Fitness!

Pankaj

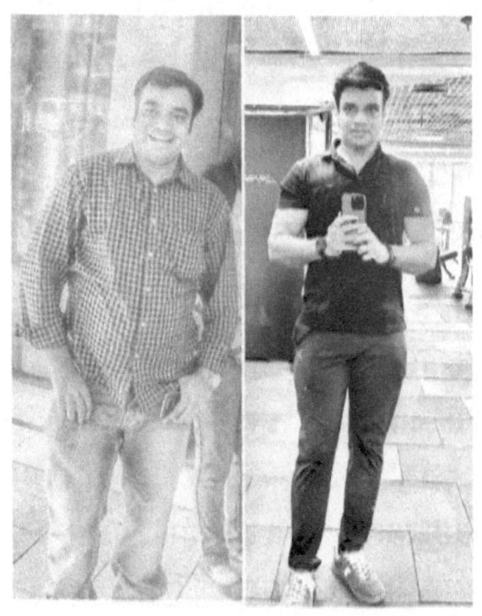

From neglecting health to embracing fitness
– my personal transformation journey

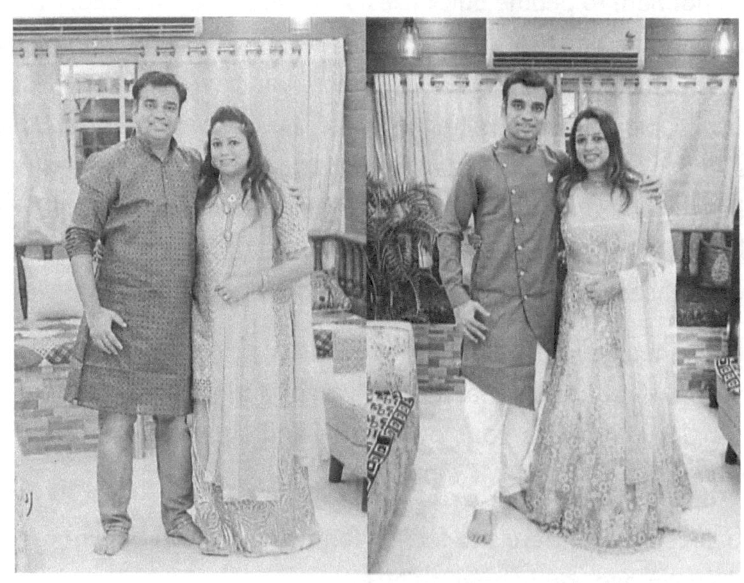

Two Diwalis apart,
same pose, same place – different we
– the difference a year of dedication can make!

HOW TO USE THIS BOOK

Welcome to *Ageless Fitness - At 40 and Beyond!* This book is designed for anyone over 40 who's ready to take charge of their fitness and well-being. Whether you're starting fresh, reigniting your routine, or striving to maintain your progress, this roadmap will guide you every step of the way.

Note: *Although this book emphasizes fitness after 40, the foundational principles of nutrition, exercise, and lifestyle habits are **universal** and applicable to all ages. If you're under 40, you'll still find valuable insights to build a strong and lasting foundation for health.*

Part 1: The Foundation

Build a strong base to support your fitness goals:

- Understand **calorie deficits** and **strength training**, the building blocks of body transformation and longevity.
- These chapters introduce essential concepts that are especially important after 40 but beneficial for all ages.

Part 2: The Essentials

Master the key lifestyle habits that amplify your results:

- Discover the importance of **sleep**, **hydration**, **lifestyle habits** and **movement** for recovery and overall performance.
- Learn sustainable practices to help you thrive physically and mentally, particularly as your body's needs change with age.

Part 3: Nutrition - Eating Smart, Not Less

Learn to fuel your body effectively at any stage of life:

- Explore the benefits of **nutrient-dense foods**, **meal planning**, **mindful eating**, and **supplements**.
- These chapters highlight the unique nutritional needs of people over 40 while offering universally relevant strategies.

Part 4: Fitness in Action: Workouts and Progress Tracking

It's time to apply your knowledge and make it personal:

- Get detailed guidance on creating **workout plans tailored to your lifestyle and goals**.
- Learn effective methods to **track your progress** and stay motivated, celebrating milestones along the way.

Whether you're a beginner or a seasoned fitness enthusiast, this section provides practical tools to fit exercise into your daily life, even with the demands of work and family.

Part 5: The Mindset

Mental resilience is key to long-term fitness:

- Develop strategies to **stay motivated**, **build habits**, and **embrace consistency**, even on challenging days.
- This section is especially relevant for those over 40, helping you stay focused as life gets busier and priorities shift.

Part 6: Debunking the Myths & Embracing the Journey

Clear up confusion and focus on what really matters:

- **Debunk fitness myths** that can derail your progress, like "carbs are the enemy" or "lifting weights makes you bulky."
- Embrace fitness as a **lifelong journey**, with insights on how your approach may evolve as you age.

Bonus Content and References

Take your fitness journey further:

- Access **practical guides**, **downloadable templates**, and **science-backed references** to keep you informed and on track.
- These resources are designed to support your unique journey, regardless of where you start.

Tips for Using This Book

1. **Start Where It Makes Sense for You**

   - While the book is structured progressively, you can jump to the sections that align with your current goals, whether that's nutrition, workouts, or mindset.

2. **Apply as You Go**

   - This isn't just a book to read - it's a guide to put into action. Use the guidelines, tips, templates, and tools to start seeing results immediately.

3. **Come Back Often**

   - Fitness is a journey, not a one-time event. Your goals and challenges will evolve, so revisit chapters as needed to adapt your approach and stay inspired.

This book celebrates the fact that **age is just a number** and that fitness is achievable at any stage of life. Whether you're over 40 or just looking to build a strong foundation, the principles in this book will help you thrive.

Now, let's get started - your healthiest self is just a page away!

INTRODUCTION

CHAPTER 1

WHY 40 IS THE NEW 30

> "Age is an issue of mind over matter. If you don't mind, it doesn't matter."
>
> **– Mark Twain**

Setting the Tone: Life Begins at 40

Welcome to your 40s - a decade that's not just about settling down, but about rising up. Gone are the days when hitting 40 meant slowing down or reluctantly embracing the 'over-the-hill' cliché. Instead, your 40s mark a new chapter filled with opportunities, strength, and self-discovery. This is your prime, where years of experience and hard-earned wisdom come together to fuel a healthier, more fulfilling life.

Remember when 40 seemed like a distant threshold where life went downhill? Fast forward, and here you are, thriving and staring at that outdated notion like it's a relic from another era. Forty isn't the end; it's a grand encore - a time to embrace your full potential with confidence, energy, and determination. You've spent decades honing your craft, balancing ambition with responsibility, and now you're ready to prioritize what truly matters: your health, happiness, and well-being.

In your 20s, life might have felt like a whirlwind of possibilities - sometimes exciting, often overwhelming. Your 30s were about finding your footing, juggling responsibilities, and beginning to understand what really matters. But now, in your 40s, you're armed with the kind of clarity that only comes from experience. This isn't about reclaiming lost youth; it's about embracing the best version of yourself, built on the foundation of everything you've learned along the way.

This is your time to focus on what truly matters. No longer tethered by the insecurities or distractions of youth, you can channel your energy into becoming the healthiest and happiest version of yourself. This journey is about self-celebration and evolution - not just in your physical fitness but in the way you live your life with purpose and passion.

So let's flip the script. Aging isn't about decline; it's about evolving. It's not about reclaiming your youth but celebrating your experience, your wisdom, and the power you've cultivated over the years. It's time to redefine what it means to be 40: strong, vibrant, and fully alive. Lace up those shoes, pick up those dumbbells, and let's dive into the best years of your life - because 40 is the new 30, and you're just getting started.

Breaking the Age Barriers: Embracing Strength and Vitality

As you enter your 40s, you might hear a barrage of perceptions about aging: "Your metabolism slows to a crawl." "Building muscle is impossible." "Exercise is risky at this age." These are not facts but misconceptions - outdated and disempowering beliefs that hold people back. Let's challenge them with science and success stories:

- **Perception 1: "Your Metabolism Slows Down Irreversibly After 40"**

  While it's true that metabolism changes with age, it's far from a "lost cause." Think of metabolism as a fire: with the right fuel and attention, it can keep burning strong. Strength training, high-intensity interval training (HIIT), and proper nutrition are powerful tools to keep it revving. Building muscle is key since muscle mass increases your resting metabolic rate, allowing you to burn calories even at rest. By maintaining muscle and staying active, you can counteract the natural slowdown.

With small, consistent efforts - such as incorporating resistance exercises into your routine or prioritizing nutrient-dense meals - you can maintain a thriving metabolic rate well into your later years. Your metabolism is not just a passive mechanism; it's adaptable and highly responsive to the positive choices you make every day.

- **Perception 2: "It's Harder to Build Muscle After 40"**

  Building muscle in your 40s is not only possible but essential. Your body might need a bit more recovery time and a targeted plan, but it's still fully capable of growing stronger. Progressive resistance training - using weights or bodyweight - combined with sufficient protein intake can work wonders. Spread your protein intake throughout the day to maximize muscle repair and growth.

Age isn't a barrier; it's a reminder to train smarter, not harder. With tailored routines and a commitment to consistency, you'll find your strength improving, whether you're lifting heavier weights, running faster, or simply feeling more energized during daily activities.

- **Perception 3: "Exercise is Too Risky When You're Older"**

  Far from being risky, exercise is a vital part of aging well. It improves mobility, reduces chronic disease risks, and enhances mental health. Focus on a mix of strength training, cardiovascular activities, flexibility exercises, and balance work to maintain your physical resilience. The biggest risk? Not exercising at all.

Even light activities like brisk walking or yoga can make a profound difference in your overall health. And as you grow more comfortable, you can gradually push your limits, discovering the incredible resilience and adaptability of your body. Exercise is not just about avoiding decline; it's about unlocking potential.

Your body is an incredible machine, capable of adapting and thriving when treated right. Fitness after 40 isn't about fighting age - It's about embracing your evolving needs and celebrating your continued strength.

Advantages of Getting Fit Now: Wisdom Meets Wellness

Harnessing Experience for Lasting Fitness

Fitness in your 40s is not about vanity or quick fixes; it's about living better, longer. With decades of life experience, you have the advantage of knowing what works for you and what doesn't.

You've tried different diets, workouts, and routines, and you're no longer swayed by fads or unrealistic promises. This is the foundation upon which you can build sustainable habits.

Your maturity also gives you a deeper appreciation for balance. You've learned to listen to your body's signals, pushing when needed and resting when necessary. This balance helps prevent injuries and keeps your fitness journey enjoyable and consistent. As a result, your efforts are more deliberate and impactful, paving the way for long-term success.

The Power of Discipline

Discipline - developed through career, family, and life challenges - is your greatest ally in fitness. In your 40s, you're more likely to set realistic goals, stick to routines, and approach setbacks with resilience. This consistency is the cornerstone of long-term success.

Beyond just sticking to a plan, you've cultivated patience - a crucial trait when it comes to achieving fitness milestones. You understand that results take time and that sustainable progress is more valuable than quick wins. This discipline and patience make you unstoppable.

The Joy of a Balanced Mindset

Perhaps the most rewarding aspect of getting fit now is the shift in perspective. Fitness is no longer about external validation; it's about feeling energized, strong, and capable. Every workout, healthy meal, and good night's sleep is an investment in your future self. By focusing on progress over perfection, you'll enjoy the journey as much as the results.

This is where wisdom meets wellness. You're not just working out to look good or counteract aging - you're building the foundation for an adventurous, fulfilling life. By embracing this balanced mindset, you're proving that the best is yet to come.

Your 40s are an invitation to rediscover yourself. This isn't just about surviving; it's about thriving, with strength, vitality, and a renewed sense of purpose. The choices you make today are not just for the present - they're for the decades of adventure, joy, and health ahead. So take that first step and keep going, because life is waiting, and it's better than ever.

Start this journey with confidence, knowing that every effort you make adds to the extraordinary life ahead. Fitness after 40 isn't just a possibility - it's an opportunity to redefine your limits and live with unparalleled vitality.

01

THE FOUNDATION

CHAPTER 2

THE GOLDEN RULE – CALORIE BALANCE

"The food you eat can be either the safest and most powerful form of medicine or the slowest form of poison."

– Ann Wigmore

Calories: What They Are & Why They Matter

A Simple Breakdown of Calories and Their Role in Your Body

Calories are a term you hear all the time - on food labels, in diet plans, and during any conversation about weight loss or nutrition. But what exactly are calories, and why do they matter so much when it comes to your health and fitness? Let's break it down in a straightforward way.

What Are Calories?

At their core, calories are units of energy. Think of calories as the fuel your body needs to function, much like how a power plant generates electricity to keep a city running. Everything you do -

whether it's thinking, walking, digesting food, or even sleeping - requires energy. This energy comes from the food and drinks you consume, which contain calories.

The foods you eat are composed of macronutrients - carbohydrates, proteins, and fats - that provide calories. Each gram of carbohydrate and protein provides about 4 calories, while each gram of fat provides about 9 calories. These calories are then converted by your body into energy, which it uses to power all its activities. Essentially, calories are your body's energy source.

The Role of Macronutrients: Protein, Carbohydrates, and Fats

Each macronutrient plays a specific and vital role in supporting your body's functions. Here's a breakdown:

- **Protein (4 calories per gram)**

    - Acts as the building block for your body.
    - Essential for repairing tissues, building and maintaining muscle, and supporting immune health.
    - Crucial for recovery after exercise and maintaining lean body mass.

- **Carbohydrates (4 calories per gram)**

    - The body's primary source of energy.
    - Fuels the brain, muscles, and other vital organs.
    - Particularly important for high-intensity activities and maintaining stamina throughout the day.

- **Fats (9 calories per gram)**

    - Vital for hormone production, cell structure, and nutrient absorption.

- o Provide a long-lasting energy source, especially during low-intensity activities or when carbohydrate stores are low.
- o Support overall brain health and help regulate body temperature.

By consuming the right balance of these macronutrients, you can fuel your body effectively, support its various functions, and achieve your health and fitness goals.

The Role of Micronutrients: Vitamins and Minerals

Micronutrients, although required in smaller quantities than macronutrients, are essential for maintaining overall health and enabling your body to function optimally.

- **Vitamins**: These are vital for processes like energy production, immune function, and cellular repair. Key examples include Vitamin D, which supports bone health; Vitamin C, which boosts immunity; and B Vitamins, which help convert food into energy. While these are some important vitamins, there are many others, each playing a unique role in keeping your body healthy.
- **Minerals**: These are crucial for structural and regulatory functions in the body. For instance, calcium strengthens bones, iron supports oxygen transport in the blood, and potassium helps regulate blood pressure and nerve function. Like vitamins, this is just a glimpse of the many essential minerals your body needs for optimal functioning.

While micronutrients don't provide calories, they are indispensable for enabling your body to utilize energy from macronutrients effectively. Consuming a variety of nutrient-dense foods - such as fruits, vegetables, whole grains, lean proteins, and healthy fats - helps ensure you meet your daily micronutrient requirements.

How Calories Work in Your Body

Imagine your body as a factory, and calories as the raw materials needed to keep production going. When you consume food, you're supplying your body with the energy it needs to operate all its machinery - from your brain to your muscles to your digestive system. This energy is necessary to keep you moving, thinking, breathing - basically, to keep you alive.

But just like a factory can only process a certain amount of raw materials at a time, your body can only use so many calories at once. The amount of calories your body needs depends on various factors, including your age, sex, weight, height, and activity level.

When you eat the right amount of calories to meet your body's energy needs, you maintain your weight. However, if you consume more calories than your body needs - more raw materials than the factory can process - the excess energy gets stored. Unlike a factory where excess materials might be set aside for later use, your body stores this extra energy as fat. It's like stockpiling raw materials in a warehouse that's already full - eventually, there's no more room, and the excess begins to accumulate, leading to weight gain.

On the other hand, if you consume fewer calories than your body needs, it starts to use the stored fat for energy, much like a factory might dip into its reserves when new raw materials are in short supply. Your body is very good at managing its energy needs, but it relies on you to provide the right amount of fuel through your diet.

The Importance of Caloric Balance

The concept of caloric balance is key to understanding weight management. Caloric balance refers to the relationship between the number of calories you consume through eating and drinking and the number of calories your body burns through all its activities. This includes not just physical exercise, but also the calories burned at rest, known as your Basal Metabolic Rate (BMR), and the calories used for digesting food, known as the Thermic Effect of Food (TEF).

Understanding this balance is crucial for managing your weight. Whether your goal is to lose, maintain, or gain weight, it all comes down to managing your caloric intake and expenditure. It's not just about the number of calories, but also about the quality of those calories - where they come from and how they nourish your body. Eating nutrient-dense foods that provide energy along with essential vitamins and minerals will help you fuel your body effectively without overloading it.

In summary, calories are not the enemy. They're a vital source of energy that your body needs to function properly. By understanding how they work and how to manage them, you can take control of your weight and overall health, ensuring that you're fuelling your body in a way that supports your goals, whether that's losing weight, maintaining your current weight, or even gaining muscle.

Finding Your Calorie Sweet Spot

Navigating the Path to Your Optimal Caloric Balance

Finding the right balance of calories for your body is like discovering the perfect rhythm in a dance. It's all about harmonizing the energy you consume with the energy you expend, creating a flow that allows you to achieve your health goals while still enjoying the process. Whether you want to maintain your current weight, shed some fat, or build muscle, understanding how to calculate and manage your caloric needs is the key to unlocking your body's full potential.

Step 1: Understanding Your Basal Metabolic Rate (BMR)

Imagine your body as a bustling city, and your Basal Metabolic Rate (BMR) is the energy required to keep the city running smoothly - even when everyone's asleep. Your BMR is the number of calories your body needs to maintain basic functions like keeping your heart beating, your lungs breathing, and your organs functioning while at rest. It's the energy required to keep the lights on, the trains running, and the infrastructure intact, even when the city seems quiet.

> *This section is all about sharing knowledge and raising awareness, so don't stress or feel overwhelmed. There are plenty of online tools that make calculating your caloric balance super simple. Just plug in a few details, and these tools will do the heavy lifting for you, helping you stay on track without any guesswork!*

Your BMR is influenced by factors like age, gender, weight, and height. For instance, a younger, taller person with more muscle mass (think of them as a larger, more vibrant city) will typically have a higher BMR than an older, shorter person with less muscle (a smaller, quieter town).

To calculate your BMR, you can use the Harris-Benedict equation, which takes these factors into account:

- **For men**:

  BMR = 88.362 + (13.397 × weight in kg) + (4.799 × height in cm) − (5.677 × age in years)

- **For women**:

  BMR = 447.593 + (9.247 × weight in kg) + (3.098 × height in cm) − (4.330 × age in years)

This equation gives you a starting point - a baseline of how many calories your body needs just to keep the essential services of your "city" running smoothly.

Step 2: Factoring in Your Activity Level

Next, we need to consider how active your "city" is throughout the day. Your Total Daily Energy Expenditure (TDEE) is like the total energy required to keep your city thriving - taking into account not just the basic functions but also the hustle and bustle of daily life.

To get a clear picture of your TDEE, you'll need to adjust your BMR based on your activity level:

- **Sedentary (little or no exercise)**: BMR × 1.2

- **Lightly active (light exercise or sports 1–3 days a week)**: BMR × 1.375
- **Moderately active (moderate exercise or sports 3–5 days a week)**: BMR × 1.55
- **Very active (hard exercise or sports 6–7 days a week)**: BMR × 1.725
- **Super active (very hard exercise or a physically demanding job)**: BMR × 1.9

Step 3: Finding Your Calorie Sweet Spot

Now comes the fun part - finding your calorie sweet spot. This is where you tailor your caloric intake to match your specific goals. Just as a well-managed city budget ensures that resources are allocated efficiently, finding your calorie sweet spot ensures that your body has the energy it needs without overloading or underfeeding it.

- **Calorie Maintenance**: If your goal is to maintain your current weight, aim to consume calories equal to your TDEE. This will ensure your body has enough energy to support all its activities without storing excess calories as fat. Imagine this as a balanced city budget - everything runs smoothly, with no deficits or surpluses.
- **Calorie Deficit for Fat Loss**: If you want to lose fat, you need to create a calorie deficit, which means consuming fewer calories than your TDEE. This is akin to a city cutting back on unnecessary expenses to pay down debt - in this case, your body uses stored fat to make up the energy shortfall. A safe and sustainable calorie deficit is usually around 500 calories per day, which can lead to losing about 1 pound (0.45 kg) of fat per week.

However, just like a city that cuts too many services can run into trouble, cutting too many calories can slow your metabolism and lead to muscle loss or nutrient deficiencies.

- **Calorie Surplus for Muscle Gain**: If building muscle is your goal, you'll need to consume more calories than your TDEE, creating a calorie surplus. Think of this as a city investing in new infrastructure to grow - your body uses the extra energy to build new muscle tissue. A surplus of 250–500 calories per day can help you gain muscle while minimizing fat gain. Focus on nutrient-dense foods that support muscle growth, such as lean proteins, healthy fats, and complex carbohydrates.

Using Tools and Resources

In today's digital world, you don't have to calculate all this on your own. There are plenty of online tools and apps that can help you find your calorie sweet spot with ease.

- Apps like **Fittr**, **MyFitnessPal**, **Cronometer**, or **Fitbit** offer personalized recommendations based on your BMR, TDEE, and activity level, making it easier to track your daily calorie intake and ensure you're staying on target.

These tools can act as your financial advisors, helping you monitor your "budget" in real-time and make adjustments as needed. They can also provide insights into the quality of your diet, offering a breakdown of macronutrients and helping you ensure that you're not just hitting your calorie goals but also getting the right balance of nutrients.

Finding Calorie Balance

Finding your calorie sweet spot is like crafting the perfect budget for your life. Spend too much (eat too many calories), and you're in debt (weight gain). Spend too little (not enough calories), and you might not have enough to cover the essentials (energy and health). The trick is finding that perfect balance where you're spending just enough to fuel your body while still saving (burning fat) for the future.

This balance is personal, just like financial planning. It's not a one-size-fits-all approach; it's about tailoring your intake to your unique needs, goals, and lifestyle. By understanding your body's caloric needs and adjusting your intake accordingly, you can take control of your weight and health, ensuring that you're fuelling your body in the most efficient and effective way possible.

Remember, the goal isn't just to hit a specific number on the scale but to find a sustainable approach that supports your long-term health and well-being. Just like a well-balanced city thrives, your body will flourish when you find and maintain that caloric sweet spot.

The Reality of "You Can't Out-Exercise a Bad Diet"

Why Exercise Alone Isn't Enough for Weight Loss or Fitness

Many people fall into the trap of thinking that as long as they're hitting the gym regularly or pushing through intense workouts, they have a free pass to eat whatever they want. After all, if you're burning calories, you should be able to indulge, right?

Unfortunately, it doesn't work that way. The reality is that exercise, while incredibly important for overall health, isn't a magic eraser for poor dietary choices. To achieve lasting weight loss or improve fitness, what you eat plays an equally crucial role.

The Calorie Equation

Let's reiterate the calorie equation. Weight management is fundamentally about the balance between **calories in** (what you eat) and **calories out** (what you burn).

- **When you consume more calories than your body needs**, the excess is stored as fat.
- **When you burn more calories than you consume**, your body taps into those fat stores for energy, leading to weight loss.

Now, exercise does burn calories, but the amount is often much smaller than you might think. For example:

- Running a mile burns roughly 100 calories.
- That's the equivalent of a single cookie or a small glass of soda.

If you're relying on exercise alone to offset high-calorie foods, you're fighting an uphill battle. It's like trying to clean up after a party by only picking up a few cups - if you don't address the mess (your diet), the room (your body) stays cluttered.

The Sinking Sand Analogy

Imagine trying to walk across a patch of sinking sand. Every step you take requires extra effort to pull your feet out of the sand and move forward.

- **Your diet is the sand.** If you're constantly eating unhealthy, high-calorie foods, it's like walking on sand that's constantly pulling you down, making every step (exercise) harder and less effective.

For example:

- After a tough workout, you might feel like you've earned a big reward, like a burger, fries, and a milkshake.
- This meal could easily add up to **1,500 calories or more.**
- To counteract that with exercise alone, you'd need to do something extreme, like running for two hours or cycling for a long distance.

Most people can't or won't do that much exercise regularly, which means the sinking sand keeps pulling them back, preventing real progress toward their fitness goals.

The Nutrient Quality Factor

Another critical aspect is the **quality of the calories** you consume. Not all calories are created equal.

- A diet rich in **whole, nutrient-dense foods** like vegetables, lean proteins, and whole grains provides your body with the essential vitamins, minerals, and nutrients it needs to function optimally.
- These foods help you feel fuller for longer, support muscle recovery, and improve your overall health.

In contrast, a diet high in processed foods, sugar, and unhealthy fats may provide plenty of calories but few nutrients. This can lead to:

- Increased hunger
- Poor energy levels
- Nutrient deficiencies

It's like trying to fuel a high-performance sports car with low-quality fuel - you might get by for a while, but eventually, it's going to affect how well the engine runs.

The Metabolic Impact

Exercise does more than just burn calories - it also has a positive impact on your metabolism. However, if your diet is full of high-calorie, low-nutrient foods, it can negate these benefits.

Consuming too much sugar and processed food can lead to:

- **Insulin resistance**
- **Inflammation**
- **Other metabolic issues**

These factors make it harder for your body to lose fat and build muscle.

The Big Picture: Sustainable Health

True fitness and health are about more than just what happens in the gym. They're about the choices you make every day:

- **What you put on your plate**
- **How you manage stress**
- **How much sleep and hydration you get**
- **How active you are overall**

Exercise is a crucial part of the equation, but it's not the whole story.

- Think of your diet as the **foundation of a house** and exercise as the structure built on top.

- A strong foundation (a healthy diet) supports everything above it. Without it, the structure is unstable and prone to collapse.

No matter how hard you train, if your diet isn't supporting your goals, you'll struggle to see the results you want.

Conclusion: Harmonizing Diet and Exercise

The reality is that **you can't out-exercise a bad diet.**

It's a hard truth, but understanding it is the first step toward making lasting changes. Exercise is an incredible tool for:

- Improving your health
- Building strength
- Enhancing your mood/

However, it works best when combined with a balanced, nutritious diet.

So, the next time you think about "earning" that extra slice of cake or pizza through a tough workout, remember the **sinking sand analogy.** Aim to solidify the ground beneath you with a healthy diet, and use exercise to enhance and complement your lifestyle - not as a way to justify poor eating habits.

When you harmonize your diet and exercise, you create a powerful duo that can lead to sustainable, long-term health and fitness.

CHAPTER 3:

STRENGTH TRAINING – WHY LIFTING WEIGHT MATTERS

"Strength is not just about muscles; it's about resilience and determination"

– Anonymous

Why Strength Training is Non-Negotiable After 40

The Essential Role of Strength Training in Aging Gracefully

As we age, the importance of maintaining our physical health becomes increasingly apparent. While cardiovascular exercise and flexibility training are vital components of a balanced fitness routine, there's one element that becomes non-negotiable after the age of 40: strength training. This isn't just about looking good in a tank top - although that's a nice bonus - it's about ensuring that your body remains strong, resilient, and capable of meeting the challenges of daily life as you grow older.

Combatting Muscle Loss: The Battle Against Sarcopenia

One of the most significant challenges we face as we age is sarcopenia, the gradual loss of muscle mass that begins in our 30s and accelerates as we hit our 40s and beyond. On average, adults can lose 3-8% of their muscle mass per decade after 30, and this rate increases even more after 60. This muscle loss isn't just about aesthetics; it has real implications for your strength, balance, and overall functionality.

Without sufficient muscle mass, everyday tasks - like carrying groceries, climbing stairs, or even standing up from a chair - can become increasingly difficult. Worse, muscle loss can lead to a vicious cycle: as you lose muscle, your metabolism slows down, making it easier to gain fat and harder to lose it. This can lead to a decline in energy levels, mobility, and overall quality of life.

But here's the good news: strength training is your secret weapon against sarcopenia. By regularly engaging in resistance exercises - whether it's lifting weights, using resistance bands, or performing bodyweight exercises - you can not only preserve the muscle you have but also build new muscle. This helps maintain your strength, keeps your metabolism revved up, and ensures that you remain capable and independent well into your later years.

Boosting Metabolism: Turning Up the Heat

Muscle tissue is metabolically active, meaning it burns calories even at rest. The more muscle you have, the higher your resting metabolic rate (RMR), allowing you to burn more calories throughout the day. After 40, metabolism slows due to hormonal changes and muscle loss, often leading to gradual weight gain despite unchanged diet and exercise habits.

Strength training counteracts this by increasing muscle mass, boosting metabolism, and making weight management easier. It's like telling Father Time, "Not so fast!" By challenging your muscles regularly, you signal your body to keep its engine running efficiently, regardless of age.

Enhancing Bone Density: Building a Strong Foundation

Strength training is vital for maintaining bone density, especially as osteoporosis risk increases with age. Weight-bearing exercises like squats and deadlifts stimulate bone growth, making bones stronger and less prone to fractures. By incorporating these exercises, you fortify your bones and create a strong foundation for overall health and mobility.

Maintaining Functional Fitness: Staying Active and Independent

Functional fitness enables you to perform daily activities with ease. Strength training improves strength, coordination, and balance, enhancing your ability to carry out tasks like lifting, sitting, and standing. Exercises like deadlifts mimic real-life movements, improving your ability to enjoy hobbies and stay independent. Additionally, it reduces fall risks, keeping you steady and confident in your movements.

Broader Health Benefits

Beyond muscle and bone, strength training offers:

- **Improved Insulin Sensitivity**: Helps regulate blood sugar and manage type 2 diabetes risk.
- **Enhanced Mental Health**: Reduces depression and anxiety, boosts cognitive function, and uplifts mood.
- **Better Sleep**: Promotes deeper, restorative sleep, supporting immune function and mental clarity.

Muscle Mass vs. Metabolism: The Great Debate

Muscle plays a key role in boosting metabolism. It's metabolically active, requiring more calories for maintenance than fat. This makes building muscle essential for maintaining a healthy RMR, which aids in weight management.

The Power of Muscle: A Calorie-Burning Furnace

Your RMR is the energy your body uses for basic functions. Muscle mass increases RMR, making it easier to maintain or lose weight. This is why strength training is a cornerstone of fitness.

Debunking Myths: Will Strength Training Make You Bulky?

Many fear that lifting weights leads to a bulky physique, but building significant muscle mass requires a specific regimen and high-calorie diet. Most people, especially women, lack the testosterone needed for this. Instead, strength training builds lean muscle, boosting metabolism and creating a toned, defined look.

The Aging Factor: Why Muscle Matters More with Age

Muscle loss accelerates with age, leading to metabolic slowdown. Strength training prevents this, keeping your metabolism active and preserving muscle mass, which is crucial for healthy aging.

Muscle Mass and Fat Loss: A Dynamic Duo

Muscle helps burn fat by increasing calorie expenditure, even at rest. Strength training also ensures weight loss comes from fat, not muscle, preserving RMR and facilitating sustainable results.

Broader Benefits

Strength training improves:

- **Bone Density**: Reducing osteoporosis and fracture risk.
- **Insulin Sensitivity**: Lowering type 2 diabetes risk.
- **Functional Fitness**: Enhancing everyday activities.
- **Injury Prevention**: Supporting joints and reducing fall risks.

Conclusion: Embrace Strength Training

Building muscle is key to maintaining metabolism and overall health as you age. Incorporate regular strength training into your routine to stay resilient and strong, no matter your age. It's time to unlock your metabolism's full potential and embrace a healthier future.

Strength training after 40 is a non-negotiable for aging well. It preserves independence, protects bones, boosts metabolism, and enhances overall well-being. Whether lifting weights or doing bodyweight exercises, the effort you invest today will pay off in a healthier, more vibrant future.

Easy-to-Follow Beginner's Guide to Strength Training

To complement the information provided in this book, a wealth of additional resources is available on the companion website. The website includes detailed guides, workout plans and tips for each of the exercise method. Whether you're looking for step-by-step instructions, variations to suit your fitness level, or tools to track your progress, the companion site is your go-to resource. It ensures you have all the support and information needed to make your fitness journey more effective and enjoyable.

A Step-by-Step Approach to Building Strength Safely and Effectively

Starting strength training might seem intimidating, especially if you're new to it or haven't lifted weights in a while. However, you don't need to become a gym rat or start with heavy barbells to reap the benefits of strength training. The key is to master the basics, focus on proper form, and progress gradually. This guide will walk you through the essential steps to get started with strength training, helping you build confidence, strength, and a solid foundation for future workouts.

Step 1: Understanding the Basics of Strength Training

Strength training involves exercises that make your muscles work against a force, typically involving resistance from body weight, free weights, resistance bands, or machines. The goal is to build muscle strength, endurance, and size while improving overall functional fitness. Before you begin, it's important to understand that strength training is about quality over quantity. Focus on mastering a few fundamental movements before moving on to more complex exercises.

Step 2: Start with Bodyweight Exercises

Bodyweight exercises are an excellent way to begin strength training because they require no equipment and can be done anywhere. These exercises help you learn proper form and build foundational strength without the risk of injury that can come from lifting heavy weights too soon.

Here are three essential bodyweight exercises to start with:

- **Squats**: Squats are one of the best exercises for building lower body strength, targeting your quads, hamstrings, glutes, and core.

How to do it:

1. Stand with your feet shoulder-width apart, toes slightly turned out.
2. Engage your core, and keep your chest up and back straight.
3. Lower your body as if you're sitting back into a chair, bending your knees and pushing your hips back.
4. Go as low as you can while keeping your back straight and knees aligned with your toes.
5. Push through your heels to return to the starting position.

Tips: Start with shallow squats if you're new, and gradually increase your depth as you get more comfortable. Aim for 2-3 sets of 10-15 repetitions.

- **Push-Ups**: Push-ups are a fantastic upper-body exercise that works your chest, shoulders, triceps, and core.

How to do it:

1. Start in a plank position with your hands placed slightly wider than shoulder-width apart.
2. Keep your body in a straight line from head to heels, engaging your core.

3. Lower your body by bending your elbows until your chest nearly touches the ground.
4. Push back up to the starting position, keeping your body straight throughout the movement.

Tips: If full push-ups are too challenging, start with modified push-ups on your knees or against a wall. Aim for 2-3 sets of 8-12 repetitions.

- **Planks**: Planks are excellent for building core strength and stability.

How to do it:

1. Start in a forearm plank position with your elbows directly beneath your shoulders and your body in a straight line from head to heels.
2. Engage your core, glutes, and quads, and hold the position without letting your hips sag or rise.
3. Hold for as long as you can while maintaining proper form.

Tips: Begin with 20-30 seconds and gradually increase your time as you build core strength.

Step 3: Progress to Weighted Exercises

Once you've mastered the basic bodyweight exercises and feel comfortable with your form, it's time to add some resistance to your routine. Incorporating weights into your workouts helps to further challenge your muscles and promote strength gains. Here are three beginner-friendly weighted exercises to try:

- **Goblet Squats**: This variation of the squat involves holding a weight (such as a dumbbell or kettlebell) close to your chest, which adds resistance and engages your upper body.

How to do it:

4. Hold a dumbbell or kettlebell close to your chest with both hands, elbows tucked in.
5. Perform a squat as described earlier, keeping the weight close to your body.
6. Push through your heels to return to the starting position.

Tips: Start with a light weight (5-10 pounds) and gradually increase as you get stronger. Aim for 2-3 sets of 8-12 repetitions.

- **Dumbbell Deadlifts**: Deadlifts are a fundamental movement that strengthens your posterior chain, including your hamstrings, glutes, and lower back.

How to do it:

1. Stand with your feet hip-width apart, holding a dumbbell in each hand in front of your thighs.
2. Hinge at your hips, keeping your back flat and shoulders back, and lower the weights toward the ground.
3. Go as low as your flexibility allows, then push through your heels to return to the starting position.

Tips: Focus on keeping your back straight and your core engaged throughout the movement. Start with lighter weights and increase as you gain confidence. Aim for 2-3 sets of 8-12 repetitions.

- **Overhead Press**: This exercise targets your shoulders, triceps, and upper chest, helping to build upper body strength.

How to do it:

1. Stand with your feet shoulder-width apart, holding a dumbbell in each hand at shoulder height, palms facing forward.
2. Press the weights overhead until your arms are fully extended, then slowly lower them back to the starting position.

Tips: Keep your core engaged and avoid arching your back during the press. Start with light weights and aim for 2-3 sets of 8-12 repetitions.

Step 4: Focus on Proper Form

Proper form is crucial in strength training to prevent injuries and ensure you're effectively targeting the right muscles. Here are some general tips for maintaining good form:

-   **Engage Your Core**: Always keep your core muscles engaged to protect your spine and maintain stability during exercises.
-   **Move Slowly and Control the Weight**: Avoid using momentum to lift weights. Focus on controlled, deliberate movements to maximize the effectiveness of each exercise.
-   **Breathe**: Don't hold your breath while lifting. Exhale during the exertion phase (e.g., lifting the weight) and inhale during the lowering phase.
-   **Watch Your Alignment**: Keep your joints aligned during exercises. For example, in squats, your knees should track over your toes, and in push-ups, your body should form a straight line from head to heels.

Step 5: Establish a Routine and Progress Gradually

When starting, it's important not to overdo it. Strength training 2-3 times per week, with at least one rest day in between sessions, is a good starting point. As you get stronger, you can gradually increase the frequency or intensity of your workouts.

As you progress, you can start increasing the weight, adding more sets or reps, and incorporating new exercises to challenge your muscles in different ways.

Day 1: Upper Body (Push & Pull)

- **Incline push-ups** – Chest & Triceps (2 sets of 8-12 reps)
- **Dumbbell rows** (or use water bottles) – Back & Biceps (2 sets of 10 reps per side)
- **Overhead dumbbell press** – Shoulders (2 sets of 8-12 reps)
- **Plank hold** – Core (Hold for 15-20 seconds, 2 sets)

Day 2: Rest or Light Activity

E.g., 20-30 minutes of brisk walking, stretching, or yoga.

Day 3: Lower Body (Legs & Core)

- **Bodyweight squats** – Quads & Glutes (2 sets of 10-12 reps)
- **Step-ups onto a sturdy chair or platform** – Legs & Glutes (2 sets of 8-10 reps per leg)
- **Calf raises (bodyweight)** – Calves (2 sets of 15 reps)
- **Side planks** – Core (Hold for 10-15 seconds per side, 2 sets)

Day 4: Rest or Light Cardio

E.g., 20-30 minutes of cycling, swimming, or a short hike.

Day 5: Full Body Strength (Push, Pull, Legs)

- **Wall push-ups or regular push-ups** – Chest & Triceps (2 sets of 8-12 reps)
- **Goblet squats** – Quads & Glutes (2 sets of 10-12 reps)
- **Bent-over dumbbell rows** – Back & Biceps (2 sets of 10-12 reps)
- **Russian twists (without weight)** – Core (2 sets of 10 twists per side)

Day 6: Active Recovery or Light Activity

E.g., 15-20 minutes of walking, stretching, or playing a casual sport.

Day 7: Rest

Focus on full recovery.

The Importance of Starting Small

Strength training 2-3 times per week is a great starting point for building a solid foundation. Rest days and light activities, such as walking or yoga, ensure your body recovers and stays active without overloading.

Remember, there are plenty of resources available to guide you, from online videos to books and fitness apps. The key is to start simple and focus on consistency. As you gain confidence, you can gradually increase weights, reps, sets, or try new exercises to keep challenging yourself. Fitness is a journey, and every step counts. Start now, stay consistent, and enjoy the progress!

Step 6: Listen to Your Body

Strength training is about pushing your limits, but it's also about respecting your body's signals. If you feel pain (not to be confused with the normal discomfort of exertion), stop the exercise and check your form. It's better to take a step back and correct any issues than to push through and risk injury.

Conclusion: Building Strength Safely and Effectively

Starting strength training doesn't require a gym membership or heavy lifting right away. By focusing on the basics - like bodyweight exercises, proper form, and gradual progression - you can build a solid foundation that will serve you well as you advance. Remember, the goal is not just to lift heavy but to lift right. With consistency, patience, and the right approach, you'll find that strength training becomes an empowering part of your fitness journey, helping you stay strong, healthy, and resilient at any age.

02

THE ESSENTIALS

CHAPTER 4

SLEEP - YOUR SECRET WEAPON

"A good laugh and a long sleep are the two best cures of anything"

– Irish Proverb

The Underrated Power of Good Sleep

Sleep is often the most overlooked component of a healthy lifestyle, yet it is arguably the most critical. While diet and exercise are essential, sleep is the glue that holds everything together, the foundation upon which your health, recovery, and overall well-being are built. Imagine trying to construct a building without a solid foundation - it might stand for a while, but eventually, it will crumble. The same is true for your body; without adequate sleep, your health, fitness, and even your mental faculties begin to deteriorate.

During sleep, your body enters a state of deep recovery and rejuvenation. It's when your muscles repair, your immune system strengthens, and your brain processes and stores memories from the day. Sleep is also the time when your body balances the critical hormones that control hunger, stress, and metabolism. For instance, leptin and ghrelin - hormones that regulate hunger and satiety - are directly affected by the quality and duration of your sleep. A lack of sleep increases ghrelin levels (which make you feel hungry) and decreases leptin levels (which signal fullness), leading to increased appetite and cravings, particularly for high-calorie, sugary foods. This hormonal imbalance not only makes it harder to maintain a healthy diet but also contributes to weight gain and other metabolic issues.

Sleep also plays a crucial role in regulating insulin sensitivity, which is essential for maintaining healthy blood sugar levels. Poor sleep can lead to insulin resistance, increasing the risk of developing type 2 diabetes over time. Moreover, inadequate sleep is linked to chronic inflammation, which is a precursor to many health problems, including heart disease, obesity, and even certain cancers.

But the impact of sleep goes beyond just physical health. Mentally, sleep is vital for cognitive functions such as memory consolidation, problem-solving, and emotional regulation. When you're sleep-deprived, your brain struggles to process information, your reaction times slow down, and your ability to make sound decisions is compromised. Emotionally, lack of sleep can lead to mood swings, increased irritability, and a higher susceptibility to stress and anxiety. In short, without sufficient sleep, your body and mind cannot function at their best, and your overall quality of life suffers.

In a world that often glorifies being busy and overworked, it's easy to fall into the trap of sacrificing sleep to get more done. However, this approach is counterproductive. The reality is that sleep is not a luxury or an afterthought - it's a necessity for optimal health and performance. If sleep were a pill, it would be the most powerful, legally available drug on the market. Prioritizing sleep is one of the most effective strategies for improving your health, enhancing your fitness results, and ensuring long-term well-being.

Sleep Cycles and Their Impact on Fitness

To fully appreciate the importance of sleep, it's essential to understand the different stages of sleep and how each one contributes to your health and fitness. Sleep is not a single, uniform state but a dynamic process that cycles through several stages, each with its own distinct functions:

1. **Light Sleep**: This is the initial stage of sleep, where your body transitions from wakefulness to a sleep state. During light sleep, your heart rate slows, your body temperature drops, and your muscles begin to relax. Although light sleep doesn't provide the deep restorative benefits of later stages, it's essential for preparing your body for more restorative sleep. Think of light sleep as the warm-up phase before a workout - it's necessary to ease your body into the deeper stages of sleep that follow.

2. **Deep Sleep (Slow-Wave Sleep)**: Deep sleep is the most restorative stage of sleep, often referred to as slow-wave sleep due to the slow brain waves that characterize it. This stage is crucial for physical recovery. It's during deep sleep that your body focuses on repairing and rebuilding tissues, strengthening the immune system, and releasing growth hormone, which is vital for muscle

repair and growth. Deep sleep is also when your body detoxifies, clearing out waste products from your brain and other organs. If you're an athlete or someone who engages in regular physical activity, deep sleep is particularly important, as it allows your body to recover from the stresses of the day.

3. **REM Sleep**: REM (Rapid Eye Movement) sleep is the stage where your brain becomes highly active, similar to when you're awake. This is the stage of sleep where most dreaming occurs, and it plays a critical role in cognitive functions such as memory consolidation, learning, and emotional processing. REM sleep is essential for mental and emotional health, helping you process the day's experiences and regulate your mood. Without adequate REM sleep, you may experience difficulties with memory, concentration, and emotional stability. It's during REM sleep that your brain processes and integrates information, making it a vital stage for learning and mental resilience.

These stages cycle throughout the night, typically repeating every 90 minutes, with each cycle becoming longer and more REM-heavy as the night progresses. The balance and progression through these stages are what make sleep restorative. If you skip out on deep or REM sleep - whether due to sleep disturbances, a poor sleep environment, or insufficient sleep duration - your body doesn't get the full benefits of rest, leaving you feeling groggy, mentally sluggish, and physically drained.

Imagine your sleep cycle as a carefully orchestrated symphony, with each stage representing a different section of instruments. Light sleep is like the wind instruments setting the tone, deep sleep is the powerful strings section driving the melody, and REM sleep is the percussion, adding rhythm and flair. If any section is missing or out of sync, the entire performance falls flat. Similarly, if you miss out on any stage of sleep, your body and mind don't function as they should, resulting in less-than-ideal performance in every aspect of your life, from your workouts to your work and personal relationships.

Practical Tips for Improving Sleep Quality

Optimizing your sleep quality is essential for reaping the full benefits of rest and recovery. Here are some practical strategies to help you create a sleep-friendly environment and establish healthy sleep habits:

1. **Establish a Consistent Bedtime Routine**: Your body's internal clock, or circadian rhythm, thrives on routine. Going to bed and waking up at the same time every day, even on weekends, helps regulate this internal clock, making it easier to fall asleep and wake up naturally. Start by establishing a calming pre-sleep routine - dim the lights, reduce noise, and engage in relaxing activities like reading, gentle stretching, or meditation. These activities signal to your body that it's time to wind down, helping you transition smoothly into sleep.

2. **Create an Optimal Sleep Environment**: Your bedroom should be a sanctuary dedicated to rest. Keep the room cool (around 15-19 degrees Celsius or 60-67 degrees Fahrenheit), quiet, and dark. A comfortable mattress and supportive pillows are essential - invest in these as you would any other health tool. Consider blackout curtains to block out light and a white noise machine

or earplugs if you're sensitive to noise. Make your bed inviting by using soft, breathable bedding. Keep the room free of distractions - reserve your bedroom for sleep and relaxation, not work or entertainment.

3. **Limit Exposure to Blue Light**: The blue light emitted by phones, tablets, and computers can interfere with your body's production of melatonin, the hormone that regulates sleep. To minimize this effect, try to avoid screens for at least an hour before bed. If this isn't possible, consider using blue light filters or special glasses that block blue light. Engage in screen-free activities before bed, such as reading a physical book, journaling, or practicing relaxation exercises.

4. **Mind Your Diet and Exercise**: What you eat and how you move during the day can significantly impact your sleep quality. Avoid large meals, caffeine, and alcohol close to bedtime, as they can disrupt your sleep. Caffeine, found in coffee, tea, chocolate, and some medications, can stay in your system for up to eight hours, making it harder to fall asleep. While alcohol might make you feel drowsy, it can interfere with your sleep cycles, particularly REM sleep, leading to a less restful night. Regular physical activity can help you fall asleep faster and enjoy deeper sleep, but try to avoid vigorous exercise close to bedtime. Instead, opt for more relaxing activities like yoga or stretching.

5. **Incorporate Relaxation Techniques**: Stress and anxiety are common culprits of poor sleep. Incorporating relaxation techniques into your bedtime routine can help calm your mind and prepare your body for sleep. Consider deep breathing exercises, progressive muscle

relaxation, or guided meditation. These practices can help reduce stress hormones and ease you into a restful state. Even simple practices like visualization - imagining a peaceful scene or mentally listing things you're grateful for - can help shift your focus from the day's worries to a more relaxed state of mind.

6. **Use Natural Sleep Aids Wisely**: If you're having trouble falling asleep despite following a good routine, natural remedies like chamomile tea, magnesium supplements, or essential oils like lavender can be helpful. Chamomile tea contains apigenin, an antioxidant that binds to receptors in your brain that promote sleepiness. Magnesium is a mineral that supports deep, restorative sleep by maintaining healthy levels of GABA, a neurotransmitter that promotes sleep. Lavender has been shown to increase slow-wave sleep, the deepest form of sleep, which helps you wake up feeling refreshed. However, these should complement, not replace, a healthy sleep routine.

7. **Monitor Your Sleep and Make Adjustments**: Pay attention to how different habits and changes affect your sleep quality. Keep a sleep diary to track your sleep patterns, including what you did before bed, how you slept, and how you felt the next day. This can help you identify patterns and make necessary adjustments. If you notice that certain activities, foods, or routines consistently disrupt your sleep, make changes to avoid them. Over time, you'll develop a personalized sleep strategy that works best for you.

8. **Stay Hydrated, but Wisely**: Hydration is important, but drinking too much liquid before bed can lead to frequent

bathroom trips during the night, disrupting your sleep. Make sure to stay hydrated throughout the day, but try to limit fluid intake in the hour or two before bed. If you do need to hydrate, opt for small sips rather than a full glass of water.

9. **Practice Patience**: Improving sleep habits takes time and consistency. You might not notice immediate changes, but stick with your new routine. Over time, you'll likely find that you fall asleep faster, sleep more soundly, and wake up feeling more refreshed and ready to take on the day.

10. **Prioritize Sleep in Your Health Routine**: Remember that sleep is just as important as diet and exercise in achieving your health and fitness goals. If you're not getting enough sleep, it will undermine your efforts in other areas. Make sleep a priority in your daily routine, and recognize that it's an essential part of your overall health strategy.

Conclusion: Prioritizing Sleep for Long-Term Success

Sleep is more than just a nightly ritual; it's the cornerstone of your health and wellness. By prioritizing sleep, you're giving your body the time it needs to recover, rebuild, and prepare for the next day. This isn't just about feeling well-rested - it's about optimizing your entire health and fitness plan. With the right sleep habits, you can enhance your physical and mental performance, improve your mood, and enjoy a healthier, more balanced life. Make sleep a priority, and watch as it transforms your health from the inside out.

The journey to better health and fitness is a marathon, not a sprint. And just like in a marathon, pacing yourself with adequate rest and recovery is key to reaching the finish line strong and resilient. So before you push harder in the gym or cut more calories from your diet, consider how well you're sleeping. It might just be the missing piece of the puzzle that takes your health and fitness to the next level.

CHAPTER 5:

HYDRATION - WATER, THE MIRACLE ELIXIR

"Pure Water is the world's first and foremost medicine"

– Slovakian Proverb

Why Staying Hydrated is Critical, Especially Now

The Essential Functions of Water in the Body

Water is far more than just a thirst quencher - it's the lifeblood of your body, involved in nearly every critical function. From the moment you wake up to the time you go to sleep, water is quietly at work, keeping you alive and well. Here's a closer look at some of the essential roles that water plays in maintaining your health:

—   **Regulating Body Temperature**: Water is crucial for maintaining a stable internal temperature. When you're hot, your body sweats, and the evaporation of sweat from your skin helps cool you down. This thermoregulation is vital, especially during intense physical activity or in hot climates. Without enough water, your body can overheat, leading to heat exhaustion or heat stroke.

— **Transporting Nutrients and Oxygen**: Every cell in your body relies on water to function properly. Water is the medium through which nutrients and oxygen are delivered to your cells. It helps dissolve vitamins, minerals, and other nutrients from the food you eat and transports them to the parts of your body that need them. Without adequate hydration, your cells can't receive the nutrients they need to perform optimally.

— **Aiding Digestion**: Water plays a key role in digestion, from saliva production to the breakdown of food in the stomach. It helps move food through your digestive tract and prevents constipation. Staying hydrated ensures that your digestive system functions smoothly, allowing your body to absorb the nutrients it needs.

— **Lubricating Joints and Protecting Tissues**: Water acts as a lubricant for your joints, helping to cushion and protect them during movement. It also protects sensitive tissues, like those in your eyes, nose, and mouth. Without enough water, your joints may feel stiff, and you might experience dry eyes or a dry mouth, which can lead to discomfort and other issues.

— **Supporting Kidney Function and Detoxification**: Your kidneys play a vital role in filtering waste products from your blood and excreting them through urine. Adequate hydration supports kidney function by helping to flush out toxins and waste products from your body. Without enough water, your kidneys have to work harder, which can lead to the buildup of waste and potentially harm your kidneys over time.

As we age, staying hydrated becomes even more critical. Our sense of thirst diminishes with age, making it easier to become dehydrated without realizing it. However, the body's need for water does not decrease. In fact, older adults are more susceptible to dehydration due to factors like reduced kidney function, medications that may cause fluid loss, and a lower overall water content in the body. Dehydration in older adults can lead to serious complications, including urinary tract infections, kidney stones, and even cognitive impairment.

Think of staying hydrated as one of the simplest, yet most powerful, health hacks you can do every day. It's a small effort that pays big dividends, especially as you age.

How Much Water Do You Really Need?

A Personalized Approach to Hydration

You've probably heard the old adage, "Drink eight glasses of water a day." While it's a decent starting point, hydration isn't one-size-fits-all. Your water needs depend on a variety of factors, including your body size, activity level, the climate you live in, and even your diet. So, how do you know if you're drinking enough water?

- **Body Weight**: Larger individuals generally need more water than smaller ones because they have more body mass to hydrate. A common guideline is to drink 35 millilitres of water for each kilogram of body weight. For example, if you weigh 72 kgs, you might aim for 2.5 litres of water per day.
- **Activity Level**: If you're physically active, especially if you're sweating, your water needs increase. You'll need extra

fluid to replace the water lost through sweat. Athletes and those who engage in regular, intense exercise may need significantly more water than sedentary individuals.
- **Climate**: Hot and humid climates increase your need for water because your body loses more fluid through sweat. Even in cooler weather, if you live at a hnb bnfcigh altitude, you might need more water due to increased respiratory fluid loss.
- **Diet**: The foods you eat can also influence your hydration needs. Diets high in protein, salt, or sugar may require more water for processing. Conversely, diets rich in water-heavy fruits and vegetables can contribute to your daily fluid intake.

Rather than focusing solely on a specific number of glasses, a better rule of thumb is to drink enough water so that your urine is pale yellow - neither too dark nor completely clear. Dark urine is a sign of dehydration, while overly clear urine may indicate overhydration.

Remember, you're not just hydrating for today - you're hydrating for the long haul. Proper hydration supports your body's functions day in and day out, helping you maintain energy, focus, and overall health.

Ways to Stay Hydrated Without Feeling Like a Camel

Making Hydration Enjoyable and Sustainable

Let's face it, drinking plain water all day can feel like a chore, especially if you're not particularly thirsty. But staying hydrated doesn't have to be a tedious task. With a little creativity, you can make hydration more enjoyable and even something to look forward to. Here are some strategies to help you stay hydrated without feeling like you're constantly chugging water:

- **Infuse Your Water**: If plain water isn't appealing, try infusing it with fruits, vegetables, and herbs. Slices of lemon, cucumber, or berries can add a refreshing flavor, while herbs like mint or basil can give your water a pleasant aroma. Not only does this make your water taste better, but it also adds a touch of elegance to your hydration routine.

- **Drink Herbal Teas**: Herbal teas are a fantastic way to increase your fluid intake, especially in cooler weather when cold water might not be as appealing. Teas like chamomile, peppermint, or ginger can be soothing and hydrating. Plus, they offer additional health benefits, such as aiding digestion or reducing stress.

- **Eat Water-Rich Foods**: Many fruits and vegetables have high water content and can contribute to your daily hydration. Foods like watermelon, cucumbers, oranges, and strawberries are not only hydrating but also packed with vitamins and minerals. Incorporating these foods into your diet is an easy and delicious way to boost your water intake.

- **Make Hydration a Habit**: Integrate hydration into your daily routine by setting reminders on your phone or using a water bottle with time markers that encourage you to drink throughout the day. Carrying a reusable water bottle with you wherever you go can also serve as a visual reminder to stay hydrated.

- **Start and End Your Day with Water**: Make it a habit to drink a glass of water first thing in the morning to kickstart your metabolism and rehydrate after a night's sleep. Similarly, end your day with a glass of water to ensure you go to bed hydrated. This simple practice can help you meet your hydration goals without much effort.
- **Experiment with Sparkling Water**: If you miss the fizz of soda, try sparkling water. It's a great way to enjoy the sensation of carbonation without the added sugars and calories of soft drinks. You can even mix it with a splash of fruit juice for a tasty, hydrating beverage.

Staying hydrated is one of the simplest, yet most effective ways to support your overall health. By incorporating these creative strategies into your routine, you can make hydration an enjoyable part of your daily life - no camel-like chugging required.

CHAPTER 6

LIFESTYLE HABITS - ELIMINATING WHAT HOLDS YOU BACK

"Fitness is more than just training and nutrition - it's about the choices you make every day. Your body is a reflection of how you treat it"

– Anonymous

When we think about fitness, we surely must focus on **calories, strength training, hydration, and sleep**. But what about the things we don't usually account for?

For many, **alcohol, smoking, stress eating, excessive caffeine, and late-night screen time** seem like small indulgences, unrelated to health and fitness. However, these habits can silently sabotage progress, slow metabolism, and interfere with recovery.

The Role of Lifestyle Habits in Fitness

Your fitness journey isn't just about what happens **inside the gym** - it's also about what happens **outside of it**. The **food you eat, your recovery habits, and even your social behaviors** all contribute to your long-term progress.

Two people can follow the **same workout plan and nutrition strategy**, but the one who manages **alcohol, smoking, stress, and sleep better** will see significantly better results.

The Chain Reaction of Lifestyle Habits on Fitness

- **Poor sleep from alcohol or screens** → Leads to low energy and cravings → Impacts workouts and recovery.
- **Smoking reduces oxygen levels** → Lowers endurance and muscle strength → Increases risk of injuries.
- **Alcohol disrupts metabolism** → Slows down fat loss and hinders muscle growth.
- **Emotional eating and caffeine dependency** → Create an endless cycle of energy crashes and poor choices.

Understanding how these factors interconnect allows you to make **better, more informed choices** - without feeling like you have to eliminate everything you enjoy.

Alcohol: Impacts Fat Loss, Muscle Growth, and Recovery

"One night of drinking might not seem like much, but its effects linger far beyond the last sip."

How Alcohol Affects Fat Burning

Many believe that as long as they work out and eat well, drinking occasionally won't hurt progress. But **alcohol has a direct impact on metabolism:**

- **Fat Burning Halts:** Your body prioritizes **breaking down alcohol** before burning fat or carbs, slowing down fat loss for up to **24–36 hours.**

- **Extra Calories Get Stored as Fat:** Alcohol is calorie-dense (**1 gram of alcohol = 7 calories**), and drinks like beer, wine, and cocktails **add hundreds of extra calories** without any nutritional benefit.
- **Increased Cravings and Overeating:** Alcohol lowers inhibitions and **increases appetite**, leading to poor food choices and excess calorie intake.

Example: A **pint of beer** (~220 calories) + **a few snacks while drinking** (~500 calories) = **a full extra meal** stored as fat.

Alcohol's Effect on Muscle Growth and Recovery

Muscle growth and recovery depend on **optimal protein synthesis, sleep, and hormone balance** - all of which alcohol interferes with:

- **Protein Breakdown Increases**: Alcohol **reduces muscle protein synthesis** by up to **37%** after a heavy drinking session.
- **Testosterone Drops, Cortisol Rises**: Alcohol lowers **testosterone** (essential for muscle repair) and increases **cortisol** (a stress hormone that promotes fat gain and muscle loss).
- **Sleep Disruption = Slower Recovery**: While alcohol may make you drowsy, it **reduces REM sleep**, leading to fatigue, poor recovery, and increased hunger the next day.
- **Smoking: Weakens Strength, Stamina, and Recovery**

*"Smoking doesn't just affect the lungs - it affects **every** part of your fitness."*

Why Smoking Lowers Endurance and Strength

Smoking reduces the body's ability to **transport oxygen efficiently**, which directly impacts cardiovascular health and muscle performance.

- **Reduced Oxygen Supply**: Less oxygen reaching the muscles means **you fatigue faster** and **struggle with endurance workouts**.
- **Weaker Muscle Strength**: Smoking **reduces blood flow to muscles**, slowing down repair and making you more prone to injury.
- **Higher Risk of Joint and Ligament Damage**: Smoking lowers **collagen production**, which weakens ligaments and tendons.

Example: Runners who smoke have a **15% lower lung capacity**, leading to slower times and faster fatigue.

Practical Steps to Cut Down and Quit

- ✓ **Start with small reductions** rather than quitting overnight.
- ✓ **Replace smoking triggers with movement** (deep breathing, a short walk, or chewing gum).
- ✓ **Increase cardiovascular exercise** to train lung efficiency.
- ✓ **Boost vitamin C intake** (helps repair oxidative damage from smoking).
- ✓ **Track your progress**, celebrating milestones to stay motivated.

Other Common Habits That Interfere with Fitness

1. Stress Eating and Emotional Snacking

- **Why it happens**: Stress triggers **cortisol**, which increases cravings for **high-sugar, high-fat foods**.

- **How it affects fitness**: Overeating - even 'healthy' foods - can still lead to **fat gain and sluggish recovery**.
- **How to manage it**:

  - Keep **nutrient-dense snacks handy** (Greek yogurt, nuts, protein bars).
  - Use **stress-relief techniques** like walking, stretching, or journaling.
  - **Stay hydrated** - thirst is often mistaken for hunger.

2. Excess Caffeine and Energy Drinks

- **Why it's an issue**: Too much caffeine increases **cortisol, affects sleep**, and causes **energy crashes**.
- **How it affects fitness**:

  - **Disrupts sleep** → Poor recovery.
  - **Overstimulates nervous system** → Increased stress.

- **Better habits**:

  - Limit caffeine to **1-2 cups per day**.
  - **Avoid energy drinks with excess sugar or stimulants.**
  - Drink **water first thing in the morning**, not just coffee.

3. Late-Night Screen Time and Poor Sleep Habits

- **Why it's a problem: Blue light from screens reduces melatonin,** making it harder to fall asleep.
- **How it affects fitness**:

  - Poor sleep **reduces muscle recovery** and increases **fat retention**.

- o Inadequate sleep leads to **increased cravings and overeating**.

- **Fix it with small changes**:

  - o **Turn off screens 1 hour before bed**.
  - o Use **blue light filters** on devices.
  - o Create a **nighttime routine** (reading, meditation, stretching).

Final Thoughts: Small Changes, Big Impact

Staying fit isn't about quick fixes or extreme sacrifices - it's about making the right choices, consistently. Smoking and alcohol don't belong in a healthy lifestyle, nor do habits like stress eating, excessive caffeine consumption, or prolonged screen time that disrupt sleep and mental well-being. These factors not only impact your energy levels but also interfere with your fitness goals, recovery, and overall health.

Your body thrives on balance - fueling it with nutritious food, getting quality sleep, managing stress effectively, and staying active. Small but intentional changes, like limiting screen exposure before bed, choosing mindful eating over emotional snacking, or replacing caffeine overload with proper hydration, can compound into significant long-term benefits.

Fitness isn't just about working out - it's about making everyday choices that support a strong, resilient body and mind. Your best self isn't built in a day, but with consistency and commitment, every decision you make brings you closer to a healthier, more vibrant life.

CHAPTER 7

THE POWER OF MOVEMENT - BEYOND THE GYM

"To move is to live. Move well, live well"

– Anonymous

Everyday Activities That Count as Exercise

When most people think about staying fit, they imagine structured workouts - lifting weights, running on a treadmill, or attending a spin class. But fitness doesn't begin and end at the gym. Daily life is full of opportunities to move, burn calories, and improve your health without formal exercise. This concept, known as Non-Exercise Activity Thermogenesis (NEAT), includes all the energy you expend during everyday activities.

NEAT is your secret weapon for staying fit effortlessly. It encompasses movements like walking to the store, playing with your kids, cleaning the house, or even fidgeting at your desk. These seemingly minor actions can add up to significant calorie burns over time, making NEAT an effective tool for weight management and overall health.

For example, the average person burns between 100 and 800 calories per day through NEAT, depending on their activity level. Tasks like standing more, doing chores, or engaging in hobbies such as gardening help increase your daily energy expenditure. It's like having a silent fitness partner working in the background, subtly supporting your health and fitness goals.

Here are some common NEAT activities and their benefits:

- **Walking:** Whether walking the dog, pacing on a call, or strolling through the park, walking is one of the simplest and most effective ways to stay active. Just 30 minutes a day can boost cardiovascular health, elevate mood, and support weight management. Choose walking over driving for short trips, or take stairs instead of elevators to add extra steps. Walking also promotes bone health and improves posture over time.

- **Gardening:** Activities like planting, weeding, and watering provide a full-body workout. Gardening strengthens muscles, improves flexibility, and reduces stress. Plus, time spent outdoors enhances mental well-being. The repetitive motions involved can help improve joint mobility, and the fresh air provides a boost to your immune system.

- **Cleaning:** Routine chores like vacuuming, scrubbing, and dusting engage multiple muscle groups and burn calories. Tackle these tasks with purpose and intensity to turn them into effective mini-workouts. For example, squatting while cleaning low surfaces can also strengthen your legs, while stretching to reach higher areas improves flexibility.

- **Climbing Stairs:** This activity elevates heart rate, strengthens legs, and improves stamina. Opt for stairs over elevators to integrate bursts of physical activity into your day. Stair climbing also enhances balance and coordination, which are critical for preventing injuries as you age.

By recognizing these everyday actions as exercise, you can embrace an active lifestyle without a formal workout routine. Even small increments of movement can accumulate into significant health benefits.

How to Stay Active Without "Working Out"

Let's face it - sometimes the idea of a structured "workout" feels overwhelming. However, staying active doesn't have to mean hitting the gym. You can incorporate movement seamlessly into your daily life with these simple strategies:

- **Take the Stairs:** An easy habit that strengthens legs and boosts cardiovascular health. It's a quick win for overall fitness. You can even challenge yourself by increasing your pace or carrying small weights to make stair climbing more intense.
- **Park Farther Away:** Choosing a parking spot farther from your destination adds extra steps to your day. Over time, this small effort makes a big difference. This strategy can also give you a chance to decompress and clear your mind before entering or leaving a busy space.
- **Walking Meetings:** Swap sedentary office meetings for walking ones. Movement improves creativity and productivity while breaking the monotony of desk work. Walking alongside a colleague also fosters more open and informal communication, enhancing collaboration.

- **Take Regular Breaks:** Prolonged sitting is detrimental to health. Combat this by standing, stretching, or taking short walks every hour. Set reminders to keep these breaks consistent. Even a quick five-minute stretch routine can improve circulation and reduce stiffness.

- **Use a Standing Desk:** Standing more throughout the day reduces health risks associated with sitting and engages your core muscles. Alternate between sitting and standing for maximum benefit. Adding a footrest or balance board can make standing more dynamic and engaging.

- **Turn Chores into Exercise:** Household tasks like vacuuming, washing the car, or scrubbing floors can double as workouts. Approach these chores with energy and intention to maximize their physical benefits. For instance, try lunging while vacuuming or using squats to reach lower areas during cleaning.

These strategies demonstrate that staying active can be simple, practical, and manageable, even on the busiest days. The key is to integrate movement naturally into your routine so that it doesn't feel like a burden.

Dance, Play, and Move: Making Fitness Fun Again

When was the last time you moved just for the joy of it? As kids, movement comes naturally through play, sports, or dancing to music. As adults, we often view exercise as a chore rather than a source of enjoyment. It's time to shift that mindset and rediscover the fun in physical activity.

Engaging in activities you genuinely enjoy makes fitness feel less like work and more like living. Here are some ideas to bring joy back to movement:

- **Dance Like Nobody's Watching:** Dancing is a fantastic cardio workout that improves coordination and burns calories. Whether in a dance class, at a party, or at home, dancing is an expressive and liberating way to stay active. Dancing can also improve mental health by reducing stress and boosting self-confidence.

- **Explore the Outdoors:** Activities like hiking, cycling, or a simple walk in the park combine physical fitness with the rejuvenating effects of nature. Outdoor movement lowers stress, boosts mood, and enhances well-being. Exploring new trails or parks can add an element of adventure and discovery.

- **Play Sports:** Team or individual sports like pickleball, basketball, soccer, badminton or tennis offer camaraderie, competition, and a fun way to stay fit. Joining a local league or playing casually with friends can keep you motivated and socially engaged. Sports also improve hand-eye coordination and agility.

- **Try Something New:** Break out of your routine by exploring new activities like martial arts, paddleboarding, or rock climbing. New challenges keep fitness exciting and engaging while improving different aspects of your health. Learning a new skill can also boost your confidence and provide a sense of accomplishment.

- **Move Mindfully:** Practices like yoga and tai chi provide a meditative approach to movement, enhancing flexibility, strength, and mental clarity. They're a great way to connect with your body and mind. Focusing on breath and controlled movements can also help manage stress and improve sleep quality.

Rediscovering the joy of movement benefits not just your physical health but also your mental and emotional well-being. Physical activity releases endorphins, reducing stress and increasing happiness. When you find activities you love, staying active becomes effortless and enjoyable.

The Key to Lasting Fitness

The best exercise is the one you enjoy and will stick with. By making movement a natural and rewarding part of your life, you can achieve lasting fitness and improved health - without the gym. So, dance, play, and move your way to a healthier, happier you!

NUTRITION - EATING SMART, NOT LESS

CHAPTER 8

NUTRIENT-DENSE FOODS AND WHY THEY MATTER

"Let food be your medicine"

– Hippocrates

When it comes to nutrition, the focus often lands on the number of calories consumed, but this approach overlooks a crucial aspect of healthy eating: nutrient density. Nutrient-dense foods provide a high amount of essential nutrients relative to their calorie content, making them the cornerstone of a healthy diet. Understanding and incorporating nutrient-dense foods into your diet is key to achieving your fitness and wellness goals without feeling deprived or restricted.

Understanding Nutrient Density

Nutrient density refers to the amount of vitamins, minerals, and other essential nutrients a food provides compared to its calorie content. In other words, nutrient-dense foods deliver more nutrients per calorie than less nutrient-dense options. This concept shifts the focus from simply counting calories to evaluating the quality of those calories - what they actually bring to the table in terms of nourishment.

For example, consider the difference between a 200-calorie serving of potato chips and a 200-calorie serving of steamed broccoli or cauliflower. The potato chips provide mostly empty calories - energy with very little nutritional value. In contrast, the broccoli/cauliflower is packed with fiber, vitamins C and K, folate, and potassium, all essential for maintaining good health. Even though both foods provide the same amount of energy, the nutrient profile of broccoli/cauliflower makes it a far superior choice for supporting overall health and well-being.

"When it comes to food, it's not just about how much you eat - it's about what you're eating. Nutrient-dense foods are like the VIPs of your diet, packing in vitamins, minerals, and other goodies without a ton of extra calories. Think leafy greens, colorful veggies, lean proteins, and whole grains. These are the foods that fuel your body and keep you feeling your best, without the empty calories."

In an Indian context, nutrient-dense options are plentiful. Consider a comparison between a plate of fried samosas and a bowl of dal (lentil soup). While the samosas might satisfy a craving, they offer little in terms of nutrition. On the other hand, dal is rich in protein, fiber, and essential minerals like iron and magnesium. It's a perfect example of a nutrient-dense food that nourishes the body without unnecessary calories.

Focusing on nutrient density allows you to maximize the nutritional value of your diet while managing calorie intake, which is particularly important for those looking to lose weight or maintain a healthy weight. By choosing nutrient-dense foods, you can eat more volume, feel fuller, and nourish your body with the nutrients it needs - all without consuming excess calories.

Examples of Nutrient-Dense Foods

Incorporating nutrient-dense foods into your diet is easier than you might think. These foods are often whole, minimally processed, and naturally rich in vitamins, minerals, and other beneficial compounds. Here are some examples of nutrient-dense foods that you can include in your daily meals:

— **Green Vegetables:** Broccoli, lettuce, green beans, and peas are packed with vitamins A, C, and K, as well as folate, iron, and calcium. These greens are also high in antioxidants, which help protect your body from oxidative stress and inflammation.

   o   In India, similar leafy greens include **methi (fenugreek leaves)**, **sarson ka saag (mustard greens)**, and **palak (spinach)**, which are rich in nutrients and commonly used in traditional dishes like palak paneer or sarson ka saag.

— **Colorful Vegetables**: Vegetables like bell peppers, carrots, sweet potatoes, and tomatoes are rich in vitamins, minerals, and phytonutrients. The vibrant colors of these vegetables indicate their high content of antioxidants, which support immune function and overall health.

   o   Indian equivalents include **gajar (carrots)**, **laal bhaji (red amaranth leaves)**, **beetroot**, and **tinda (Indian round gourd)**. These vegetables are often used in salads, sabzis, and other traditional Indian recipes.

- **Berries**: Blueberries, strawberries, raspberries, and blackberries are not only delicious but also loaded with fiber, vitamin C, and powerful antioxidants like anthocyanins. Berries are low in calories but high in nutrients, making them a perfect snack or addition to smoothies and salads.

  - In India, you might consider **amla (Indian gooseberry)**, which is exceptionally high in vitamin C and antioxidants. **Jamun (black plum)** and **mulberry** are other nutrient-dense fruits available seasonally and used in various traditional remedies and dishes.

- **Lean Proteins**: Foods like chicken breast, turkey, lean cuts of beef, tofu, and legumes provide high-quality protein without excessive fat or calories. Protein is essential for muscle repair, growth, and overall body function.

  - Indian diet staples like **dal (lentils), chana (chickpeas), paneer (Indian cottage cheese)**, and **moong dal (mung beans)** are excellent sources of plant-based protein. **Fish like rohu and hilsa**, common in Indian cuisine, also provide lean protein and omega-3 fatty acids.

- **Whole Grains**: Brown rice, quinoa, oats, and whole wheat products are rich in fiber, B vitamins, and important minerals like magnesium and iron. Whole grains provide sustained energy and support digestive health.

  - In the Indian context, **jowar (sorghum), bajra (pearl millet), ragi (finger millet)**, and **whole wheat atta**

(flour) used for making chapatis are examples of whole grains that are nutrient-dense and form the base of many traditional Indian diets.

- **Nuts and Seeds**: Almonds, walnuts, chia seeds, and flaxseeds are excellent sources of healthy fats, protein, and fiber. They also contain important nutrients like vitamin E, magnesium, and omega-3 fatty acids, which support heart health and brain function.

  o Indian varieties include **almonds (badam)**, **cashews (kaju)**, **sesame seeds (til)**, and **flaxseeds (alsi)**. These are commonly consumed as snacks or used in dishes like laddoos, chutneys, and curries.

- **Fatty Fish**: Salmon, mackerel, sardines, and trout are rich in omega-3 fatty acids, protein, and vitamin D. Omega-3s are crucial for heart health, reducing inflammation, and supporting cognitive function.

  o In India, **rohu**, **hilsa**, and **mackerel (bangda)** are popular fatty fish rich in omega-3s. They are often prepared in traditional dishes like Bengali mustard fish curry or Goan fish curry, providing both taste and nutrition.

By incorporating a variety of these nutrient-dense foods into your diet, you ensure that your body gets a wide range of nutrients necessary for optimal health.

How Nutrient-Dense Foods Support Fitness Goals

Nutrient-dense foods play a vital role in supporting your fitness and wellness goals, whether you're aiming to build muscle, lose weight, or simply maintain a healthy lifestyle. These foods provide the essential nutrients your body needs to perform at its best, both in and out of the gym.

1. **Fuelling Workouts**: Nutrient-dense foods provide the energy and nutrients necessary to fuel your workouts. For example, complex carbohydrates from whole grains and vegetables supply a steady source of energy, while lean proteins help repair and build muscle tissue. Consuming a nutrient-rich meal before and after exercise ensures that your body has the fuel it needs to perform and recover effectively.

   o   In India, meals like a **banana with a handful of nuts, a slice of whole-grain toast with peanut butter, or a bowl of yogurt with fruit** can provide the quick energy you need to sustain your exercise routine. These options are rich in easily digestible carbs and moderate protein, making them ideal for fuelling your workout and aiding recovery.

2. **Supporting Recovery**: After a workout, your body needs to replenish glycogen stores and repair muscle fibers. Nutrient-dense foods like lean proteins, healthy fats, and antioxidant-rich fruits and vegetables play a critical role in this recovery process. They help reduce inflammation, repair damaged tissues, and restore

energy levels, allowing you to bounce back stronger for your next workout.

- o   A post-workout meal in the Indian context could include **paneer bhurji with whole wheat toast**, a **smoothie with curd, spinach, and banana**, or a **simple dal-roti** combination, providing the necessary nutrients for muscle repair and recovery.

3. **Enhancing Metabolism**: A diet rich in nutrient-dense foods can help enhance your metabolism. Foods high in protein, for instance, have a higher thermic effect, meaning your body burns more calories digesting and metabolizing them compared to fats or carbohydrates. Additionally, foods rich in fiber, like whole grains and vegetables, support digestive health and help regulate blood sugar levels, both of which contribute to a healthy metabolism.

- o   Indian foods like **idli with sambar, oats upma**, or a **sprout salad** can boost your metabolism while providing sustained energy throughout the day. These dishes are not only filling but also help regulate digestion and blood sugar levels.

4. **Promoting Satiety**: One of the challenges in managing weight is controlling hunger and preventing overeating. Nutrient-dense foods, particularly those high in fiber and protein, help you feel fuller for longer, reducing the likelihood of overeating. This is because these foods slow down digestion and stabilize blood sugar levels, preventing the energy crashes that can lead to cravings for unhealthy snacks.

- o Traditional Indian dishes like **dal-chawal (lentils with rice), roti with sabzi,** or a **bowl of curd with fruits and seeds** are perfect examples of meals that promote satiety. They keep you full and satisfied, reducing the temptation to snack on less healthy options.

5. **Preventing Nutrient Deficiencies**: Nutrient-dense foods ensure that your body gets the vitamins, minerals, and other essential nutrients it needs to function properly. Deficiencies in key nutrients can lead to fatigue, weakened immune function, and impaired performance, all of which can hinder your fitness goals. By focusing on nutrient-dense options, you provide your body with the tools it needs to stay healthy and perform at its best.

   - o Indian staples like **dal (lentils), green leafy vegetables (like palak and methi), curd**, and **nuts** ensure that you get a rich supply of nutrients that support overall health and wellness.

It's important to recognize that achieving a nutrient-dense diet doesn't require relying on expensive, imported, or trendy foods often marketed as "superfoods." Locally available foods, rooted in regional cuisines and traditions, offer an abundance of affordable and nutrient-rich options. Staples like whole grains, lentils, fresh vegetables, fruits, nuts, and seeds often provide all the essential nutrients your body needs to thrive.

By embracing locally sourced, seasonal, and traditional ingredients, you can create balanced, delicious meals that support your health without straining your budget. Good nutrition is not about exotic or costly foods - it's about making smart, sustainable choices from what's accessible and aligned with your cultural and dietary preferences.

CHAPTER 9

ART OF SMART AND SIMPLE MEAL PLANNING

"By failing to prepare, you are preparing to fail"

– Benjamin Franklin

> **Note:** Dietary preferences vary - whether you follow a vegetarian, non-vegetarian, vegan, or other diet, quantified nutrition can be adapted to suit your needs. While the sample meal plans mention specific food items, there are suitable replacements for every ingredient based on individual preferences. **A detailed food substitution chart is available on the companion website to help tailor meal plans to your macronutrient requirements.**

The Importance of Quantified Nutrition

In today's fast-paced world, it's easy to overlook the importance of planning our meals with precision. However, when you're striving to meet specific health and fitness goals - whether it's losing weight, building muscle, or maintaining overall wellness

- quantified nutrition becomes a key component of success. Quantified nutrition involves understanding and managing the amounts of calories and macronutrients - proteins, carbohydrates, and fats - you consume, ensuring that your diet is aligned with your goals.

Just as we quantify other aspects of our lives - whether it's money, time, or performance - why should our nutrition be any different? Food is the fuel that powers our bodies, so it's crucial that we measure and manage it with the same care we would apply to anything else important in our lives. By quantifying your nutrition, you can ensure that your body receives the exact amount of calories and nutrients it needs to function optimally, achieve your goals, and maintain your health.

Quantification: Calorie & Macronutrient Balance

1. Understanding Your Caloric Needs:

The foundation of quantified nutrition lies in understanding your daily caloric needs. This is determined by factors such as your age, gender, weight, activity level, and fitness goals. For instance, if you're aiming to lose weight, you'll want to consume fewer calories than your body requires to maintain its current weight, creating a calorie deficit. If you're focused on building muscle, you may need a slight calorie surplus to provide the extra energy required for muscle growth.

To calculate your daily calorie needs, you can use an online Total Daily Energy Expenditure (TDEE) calculator, which takes into account your Basal Metabolic Rate (BMR) and your activity level.

Once you have your TDEE, you can adjust your calorie intake based on your goals.

For example, if your TDEE is 2,200 calories and you're aiming for weight loss, you might aim for a daily intake of 1,700-1,900 calories to create a sustainable deficit. This deficit should be modest to prevent feelings of extreme hunger or fatigue, which can make it difficult to stick to your plan.

2. Measuring Raw Ingredients for Accuracy:

When quantifying your meals, it's essential to measure ingredients in their raw form. Measuring raw food before cooking allows for accurate tracking of calories and macronutrients, as cooking can alter the weight and volume of foods. A basic kitchen scale is an invaluable tool for this purpose. By measuring ingredients like raw rice, cooking oil, or vegetables, you can ensure that you're consuming the exact quantities needed to meet your caloric and nutritional goals.

For example, if you plan to eat 100 grams of rice, you would measure it on the scale before cooking. After cooking, the weight of the rice will increase due to water absorption, but the nutritional content remains based on the raw weight. This practice eliminates the guesswork and ensures that your diet is precisely aligned with your objectives.

3. Balancing Macronutrients:

Once you know your calorie target, the next step in quantified meal planning is determining the right balance of macronutrients - proteins, carbohydrates, and fats. As discussed in Chapter 2, each macronutrient plays a specific role in your body:

1. **Protein**: Essential for muscle repair and growth, protein should make up about 25-30% of your total daily calories if you're focusing on fitness goals. For a 1,800-calorie diet, this equates to approximately 113-135 grams of protein per day. Indian sources of protein include **dal (lentils), soya, paneer, chickpeas, eggs**, and **fish like rohu**.

2. **Carbohydrates**: Carbohydrates provide the energy needed for daily activities and workouts. Depending on your goals, 40-50% of your daily calories should come from carbs. For an 1,800-calorie diet, this translates to around 180-225 grams of carbohydrates. Choose complex carbs like **brown rice, quinoa, bajra, jowar, whole wheat**, and **millets** for sustained energy.

3. **Fats**: Healthy fats are necessary for hormone production and overall cell function. They should constitute about 20-30% of your daily calories, which means 40-60 grams of fats per day for an 1,800-calorie diet. Include sources like **ghee, nuts, seeds, olive oil, and fatty fish**.

4. **Cooking Fats**: It's also important to account for the fats you use in cooking. Commonly used fats like oil, ghee, and butter should be measured to ensure they fit within your daily caloric budget. For instance:

5. 5 grams of ghee or butter (1 teaspoon) = 45 calories, 5 grams of fat

6. 5 grams of olive oil (1 teaspoon) = 40 calories, 4.5 grams of fat

Measuring these ingredients before cooking is key to maintaining your nutritional balance. For example, if you're using 10 grams of ghee to prepare dal, that's an additional 90 calories and 10 grams of fat to factor into your meal.

By balancing these macronutrients according to your specific needs, you can ensure that your body is getting the right fuel for both performance and recovery.

Practical Tips for Quantified Meal Planning

1. **Set Your Goals and Track Your Intake**: Start by setting clear goals - whether it's fat loss, muscle gain, or maintenance. Use a food tracking app or a simple journal to record your daily intake. This helps you stay accountable and ensures that you're hitting your calorie and macronutrient targets. For example, if your goal is to consume 120 grams of protein daily, you can track how much you're getting from sources like **dal, paneer, chicken**, or **fish** throughout the day.

2. **Plan Your Meals with Precision**: Plan meals that align with your macronutrient needs. For example, a breakfast of **masala oats** with **curd** provides a good balance of protein and carbs, while a lunch of **grilled chicken or paneer salad** with a whole wheat chapati ensures you're getting a mix of protein, complex carbs, and healthy fats. Use kitchen scales and measuring cups to ensure you're accurately portioning your food, including cooking fats like ghee or oil.

3. **Batch Cook and Portion Wisely**: To save time, batch cook staple foods like **rice, brown rice, quinoa, grilled chicken, or dal** and portion them into individual servings that meet your macronutrient targets. For instance, cook a batch of **dal tadka** and portion it into containers, each providing 15-20 grams of protein. Don't forget

to measure the cooking oil or ghee used during the preparation, as it contributes to your daily fat intake.

4. **Include Macronutrient-Rich Snacks**: Snacks are an important part of your diet, especially if they contribute to your overall macronutrient intake. Choose snacks that align with your goals, such as **Greek yogurt with flaxseeds** for a protein boost or **almonds and walnuts** for healthy fats. For a carbohydrate-rich snack, try **fruits like bananas or poha**.

5. **Customize Based on Activity Level**: Your macronutrient needs might vary based on your activity level. On workout days, you may require more carbohydrates to fuel your exercise and more protein to support recovery. Plan your meals accordingly - on days when you have an intense workout planned, increase your intake of **carb-rich foods like sweet potatoes, whole wheat roti, or oats** to ensure your muscles are adequately fuelled.

6. **Monitor and Adjust**: Quantified meal planning isn't a one-time task. Regularly monitor your progress and adjust your plan as needed. If you're not seeing the results you want, you may need to tweak your calorie intake or macronutrient balance. For instance, if you're feeling sluggish during workouts, you might need to increase your carb intake slightly. Alternatively, if you're not seeing the desired weight loss, you might need to adjust your calorie deficit.

Sample Quantified Meal Plan for a Busy Week

Here's a sample meal plan that aligns with quantified nutrition principles, designed to provide approximately 1,800 calories with a balanced distribution of macronutrients. All measurements are for raw ingredients, ensuring accurate tracking of calories and nutrients, including the use of cooking fats.

> *This sample meal plan is designed to illustrate quantified nutrition in action. Food choices can be adjusted based on your dietary preferences - vegetarian, non-vegetarian, vegan, or otherwise. You can refer to the companion website for detailed food substitution charts and customizable meal planning templates to help you create a plan tailored to your macronutrient needs.*

Day 1 Meal Plan

Meal	Item	Protein (g)	Carbs (g)	Fats (g)	Calories
Breakfast	50g raw oats	6	30	3	190
	100ml low-fat milk	3	5	1.5	50
	15g almonds	3	2	8	90
	10g honey	0	8	0	30
Total		12g	50g	15g	350
Lunch	150g raw chicken breast (grilled)	33	0	3.5	165
	100g raw mixed greens	2	5	0	25
	50g cucumber	0	2	0	8
	50g carrots	0	5	0	20
	20g lemon-yogurt dressing	1	3	1	20
	30g whole wheat chapati (raw)	3	20	0.5	100

Meal	Item	Protein (g)	Carbs (g)	Fats (g)	Calories
	5g oil (for cooking)	0	0	5	45
Total		**35g**	**40g**	**15g**	**450**
Dinner	50g raw dal (cooked as dal tadka)	12	30	1	170
	50g rice (uncooked)	4	40	0	180
	50g spinach (cooked)	2	4	0	20
	100g curd	4	5	2	50
	10g ghee (for cooking)	0	0	10	80
Total		**25g**	**60g**	**18g**	**500**
Snack	25g almonds	6	3	14	160
	100g apple	0	22	0	40
Total		**5g**	**25g**	**10g**	**200**
Daily Total		**77g**	**175g**	**58g**	**1,800**

Day 2 Meal Plan

Meal	Item	Protein (g)	Carbs (g)	Fats (g)	Calories
Breakfast	50g raw oats	6	30	3	190
	100ml low-fat milk	3	5	1.5	50
	15g almonds	3	2	8	90
	10g honey	0	8	0	30
Total		**12g**	**50g**	**15g**	**350**
Lunch	100g raw paneer (cooked as bhurji)	18	5	16	220

Meal	Item	Protein (g)	Carbs (g)	Fats (g)	Calories
	60g whole wheat chapati (raw)	6	40	1	180
	100g cucumber	0	4	0	16
	5g ghee (for cooking)	0	0	5	45
Total		**25g**	**50g**	**15g**	**450**
Dinner	100g raw mackerel (fish curry)	20	0	10	160
	50g quinoa (uncooked)	7	40	2	200
	100g mixed vegetable stir-fry	3	10	0.5	50
	5g olive oil (for cooking)	0	0	5	45
Total		**30g**	**45g**	**12g**	**450**
Snack	100g curd	4	5	2	50
	10g flaxseeds	2	4	4	50
	50g mixed berries	1	20	1	60
Total		**10g**	**30g**	**7g**	**200**
Daily Total		**77g**	**185g**	**49g**	**1,800**

This meal plan is designed to be flexible and adaptable, allowing you to make adjustments based on your personal needs and preferences. The key is consistency - tracking your intake and making informed choices that align with your macronutrient targets. By approaching nutrition with intention and precision, you empower yourself to take control of your health, fuel your body optimally, and set yourself up for long-term success.

In today's fast-paced world, it's easy to overlook the importance of planning meals with precision. Yet, when it comes to achieving specific health and fitness goals - whether it's losing weight, building muscle, or maintaining overall wellness - quantified nutrition plays a crucial role. Just as we carefully track our finances, time, or performance, why should our nutrition be any different?

Remember, food is the fuel that powers our bodies, and managing it with the same level of attention ensures that we meet our goals effectively.

CHAPTER 10

ENJOYING YOUR FOOD SOJOURNS

"Savor the flavour, and enjoy the journey"

– Anonymous

Maintaining your nutrition goals doesn't mean you have to sacrifice your lifestyle or miss out on enjoying your favorite foods during special occasions like travel, festivals, or parties. Quantified nutrition provides you with a scientific approach to balance and moderation, allowing you to enjoy your food while staying within your caloric budget. Here's how you can seamlessly integrate your nutrition goals with the joy of special occasions, without feeling deprived or guilty, illustrated with practical, real-life examples.

Strategic Planning and Balancing Meals

Strategic planning is a powerful tool that enables you to enjoy special occasions without compromising your nutritional goals. By making thoughtful, calculated decisions throughout the day, you can indulge in festive meals while keeping your overall calorie intake in check.

- **Planning Ahead**: Imagine you've been invited to a wedding reception in the evening, and you know there will be a lavish spread of rich foods - think **paneer butter masala, biryani, and gulab jamun**. Instead of worrying about the calories, plan your day's meals accordingly. Start with a high-protein, low-carb breakfast like **scrambled eggs with spinach**. For lunch, opt for something light but filling, such as a **sprouts salad or grilled chicken salad** with lots of greens and a light lemon vinaigrette.

By doing this, you save a significant portion of your daily calorie allowance for the evening, giving you the flexibility to enjoy the wedding feast without guilt. This approach allows you to partake in the celebration, savor the dishes you love, and still stay within your caloric budget.

- **Balancing Treats with Healthy Choices**: Let's say you're attending a Diwali party, and you know you'll be tempted by **mithai** (Indian sweets) like **ladoos and kaju katli**. Instead of depriving yourself, plan to have smaller portions of these sweets. For instance, if you love **kaju katli**, have one piece and savor it slowly. Balance this indulgence by eating lighter, nutrient-dense meals throughout the rest of the day.

For breakfast, you might have a bowl of **oats topped with fruit** and a sprinkle of nuts. For lunch, a bowl of **dal with steamed vegetables** can provide the nutrients you need without adding too many calories. This way, you can enjoy your favorite Diwali treats in moderation without derailing your nutrition goals.

- **Strategizing for Specific Occasions**: Suppose you're traveling to a destination known for its rich cuisine, like

Amritsar, famous for its **amritsari kulchas and lassi**. Instead of avoiding these local delicacies, plan your meals strategically. Start your day with a light breakfast, perhaps **yogurt with a handful of nuts**, and skip heavy snacks in the morning. When it's time to indulge in an **amritsari kulcha**, enjoy it mindfully, and balance it out by having a lighter meal for dinner, such as a **soup or a simple salad**.

This way, you get to experience the local cuisine without going overboard. The key is not to restrict yourself but to balance indulgent meals with lighter, more nutritious options.

Mindful Eating and Portion Control

Mindful eating and portion control are essential for enjoying your favorite foods during special occasions without overindulging. These practices help you savor your meals while keeping your calorie intake in check.

- **Portion Control**: Consider a scenario where you're at a family gathering, and there's a buffet with an array of dishes – **paneer tikka, butter chicken, naan, biryani, and an assortment of desserts**. Instead of loading up your plate, use a smaller plate and take a little bit of everything you want to try. For example, take a small piece of **naan**, a few spoonfuls of **paneer tikka or butter chicken**, and a small portion of **biryani**.

When it comes to desserts, if you're eyeing the **gulab jamun**, take just one piece and savor it. This way, you get to enjoy all the flavors of the meal without overloading on calories. Portion control allows you to indulge in your favorite foods without feeling deprived or guilty afterward.

- **Mindful Eating**: Imagine you're at a festival, like Eid, where the table is filled with rich dishes such as **biryani, kebabs, and sheer khurma**. Instead of rushing through your meal, practice mindful eating. Take small bites, chew slowly, and focus on the flavors and textures of each dish. For instance, as you eat the **kebabs**, pay attention to the spices and the tenderness of the meat.

By eating mindfully, you're more likely to notice when you're full, which prevents overeating. This practice not only enhances your enjoyment of the meal but also helps you maintain control over your calorie intake.

- **Staying Hydrated**: Let's say you're attending a summer party, and it's hot outside. The event is outdoors, and there's a bar offering a variety of alcoholic drinks. Instead of reaching for a cold beer, start with a glass of water or a fresh lime soda. Drinking water before and during meals helps you feel full and reduces the chances of overeating.

If you decide to have a drink, alternate between alcoholic beverages and water. For example, after a glass of wine, drink a glass of water before having another. This simple strategy not only keeps you hydrated but also helps manage your overall calorie intake, as alcoholic drinks can be surprisingly high in calories.

Focusing on the Experience Beyond Food

While food is often a central part of social events, shifting your focus to the experience beyond eating can help you enjoy the occasion more fully. Engaging in the social and emotional aspects of the event can reduce the temptation to overeat and help you appreciate the celebration in its entirety.

- **Engaging in Activities**: Imagine you're at a wedding reception with a dance floor and live music. Instead of lingering at the buffet, get involved in the activities. Join the dancing, participate in traditional rituals, or simply mingle with other guests. Dancing not only adds to the fun but also burns calories, helping to offset some of the indulgent foods you might have eaten.
- **Social Interaction**: Picture yourself at a holiday party where the focus is on socializing and catching up with loved ones. Engage in conversations that naturally slow down your eating pace. For instance, if you're enjoying a piece of cake, take small bites while chatting with a friend. This gives your body time to register fullness, helping you avoid the temptation to go back for seconds.
- **Appreciating the Atmosphere**: Imagine you're celebrating Holi, surrounded by vibrant colors, music, and joy. Instead of making food the centerpiece of your day, take in the atmosphere. Enjoy the colors, participate in the fun, and let the celebration itself be the highlight. When it's time to eat, approach the meal with mindfulness.
- **The Science of Balance: Enjoying Food Without Sacrificing Health**

Quantified nutrition doesn't mean you have to sacrifice the goodness of your food or your favorite treats. Instead, it offers a golden trade-off - allowing you to enjoy all the flavors and experiences you love while staying healthy and within your caloric budget. Here's how you can enjoy life's special moments without compromising your health goals, with practical examples:

- **Indulgence Doesn't Mean Overindulgence**: You can still enjoy the foods you love; it's all about moderation. A well-planned approach allows you to indulge without guilt, knowing that your overall nutritional balance remains intact. For instance, if you're at a friend's birthday party and there's a delicious chocolate cake, have a small slice and savor it. Enjoy the treat for what it is - a special occasion dessert. The next day, return to your regular eating habits, knowing that one indulgent moment hasn't derailed your progress.
- **Flexibility in Nutrition**: Life is full of unexpected events and celebrations, and your nutrition plan should be flexible enough to accommodate these. For example, if you're unexpectedly invited to a lunch out with colleagues, choose wisely from the menu. Opt for grilled or baked dishes, ask for dressings on the side, and skip the extra bread or dessert if you've already indulged earlier in the week. This flexibility ensures you can participate in social events without feeling restricted or guilty.
- **Empowerment Through Knowledge**: Quantified nutrition empowers you with the knowledge to make informed decisions about your food. It's not about saying no to your favorite dishes, but rather about understanding how to enjoy them in a way that aligns with your goals. For example, if you know a traditional **curry** is high in calories, you can balance it out by choosing a smaller portion and pairing it with a side of vegetables instead of rice. This way, you still enjoy the dish without exceeding your calorie goals.

In conclusion, the beauty of quantified nutrition lies in its ability to blend structure with flexibility, allowing you to enjoy the richness of life's moments - whether it's a festival, a family gathering, or a holiday - without losing sight of your health goals. By planning ahead, practicing mindful eating, and focusing on the experience beyond food, you can maintain your nutritional integrity while fully enjoying every celebration. Through strategic planning, mindful portion control, and appreciating the experience beyond food, you can savor every moment of life's special occasions without compromising your commitment to health and wellness.

CHAPTER 11

DECODING NUTRITION LABELS

"The most important classroom is your kitchen – nutrition labels are your textbooks"

– Anonymous

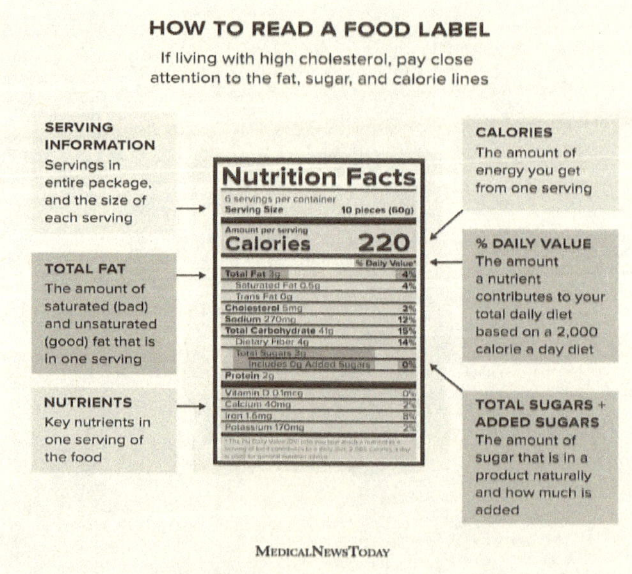

Figure 1: Sample Nutrition Label

In today's fast-paced world, where convenience often trumps careful consideration, understanding nutrition labels is more crucial than ever. These labels are your window into the nutritional content of the foods you consume, offering valuable insights that can help you make healthier choices. Whether you're managing your calorie intake, monitoring sugar consumption, or increasing your protein intake, nutrition labels provide the information you need to align your eating habits with your health goals.

Breaking Down the Nutrition Label

At first glance, a nutrition label can seem overwhelming, but breaking it down into its key components makes it much easier to understand. Here's a detailed look at what each part of the label tells you:

- **Serving Size**: The serving size is the foundation for everything else on the label. It tells you the recommended amount for consumption and sets the stage for all the nutritional information that follows. It's essential to note that the serving size listed might be smaller or larger than what you actually consume. For example, if the serving size is 1 cup and you eat 2 cups, you'll need to double all the numbers on the label to reflect your actual intake.

- **Calories**: Calories indicate the amount of energy you'll get from a serving of this food. Understanding this number is critical if you're tracking your daily caloric intake. Remember, if the serving size is small and you're likely to eat more, the total calories can add up quickly.

- **Macronutrients**: The macronutrients section covers fats, carbohydrates, and proteins, each of which is broken down further:

- **Fats**: Includes total fat, saturated fat, and sometimes trans fats. Fats are essential for health, but the type of fat matters. Saturated fats should be consumed in moderation, while trans fats should be avoided whenever possible.
- **Carbohydrates**: Listed as total carbohydrates, this includes dietary fiber and sugars. Fiber is beneficial for digestion and helps regulate blood sugar, while sugars (especially added sugars) should be consumed sparingly.
- **Proteins**: Essential for muscle repair and overall body function, protein should be a staple in your diet. The amount listed here can help you determine if the food meets your protein needs.

- **Micronutrients**: These include vitamins and minerals like Vitamin D, calcium, iron, and potassium. Although they appear in smaller amounts compared to macronutrients, they are vital for overall health and should not be overlooked.

Understanding these components allows you to evaluate how a food fits into your overall diet, ensuring you meet your nutritional needs without exceeding your caloric budget.

Understanding Daily Value Percentages

The % Daily Value (%DV) helps you understand how much a nutrient in a serving of food contributes to your total daily diet, based on a 2,000-calorie diet - a standard benchmark. However, your individual needs might vary depending on factors like age, gender, activity level, and health goals.

- **Low vs. High**: A %DV of 5% or less is considered low, which might be beneficial for nutrients like saturated fat or sodium that you're trying to limit. On the other hand, a %DV of 20% or more is considered high, which can be advantageous for nutrients like fiber or vitamins that you want to increase.
- **Personalized Application**: If you're aiming to reduce your intake of certain nutrients, such as added sugars or sodium, look for foods with lower %DVs in these areas. Conversely, if you're trying to boost your intake of beneficial nutrients like fiber or calcium, seek out foods with higher %DVs.

Using %DVs helps you quickly assess whether a food is a good choice for your dietary needs and can guide you in balancing your overall nutrient intake throughout the day.

Identifying Hidden Sugars and Fats

One of the trickiest parts of reading nutrition labels is identifying hidden sugars and unhealthy fats, which are often disguised under different names or buried in the ingredient list.

- **Hidden Sugars**: Sugars can go by many names on a label - high fructose corn syrup, sucrose, glucose, dextrose, and more. These added sugars contribute to excess calorie intake without providing essential nutrients. Be mindful of the total sugars listed on the label, and check the ingredients list for hidden sources of added sugars.
- **Unhealthy Fats**: Trans fats, often listed as "partially hydrogenated oils," are particularly harmful and should be avoided entirely. Even if the label lists 0 grams of trans fats, it's wise to scan the ingredients list, as products can

contain up to 0.5 grams per serving without declaring it on the label.

By being aware of these hidden ingredients, you can avoid foods that may derail your health goals, even if they appear healthy at first glance.

Serving Sizes and Portion Control

Serving sizes on nutrition labels are often smaller than what people typically eat, which can lead to underestimating your calorie and nutrient intake.

- **Realistic Portions**: It's important to compare the serving size on the label to the portion you actually consume. For instance, if a serving of cereal is ¾ cup but you typically pour 2 cups into your bowl, you're consuming nearly three times the calories and nutrients listed.
- **Portion Control Tips**: To better manage portion sizes, consider measuring your food until you become familiar with what a standard serving looks like. Using a kitchen scale to measure raw food can help ensure accuracy. Understanding portion sizes helps you stick to your nutritional goals without the risk of unintentional overeating.

This awareness can help you make more informed decisions about how much you're really consuming and adjust your portions to better align with your dietary goals.

Using Labels to Make Healthier Choices

Nutrition labels are a powerful tool for comparing products and making healthier choices, whether you're shopping at the grocery store or dining out.

- **Comparison Shopping**: When faced with multiple options, use the nutrition labels to compare calories, fats, sugars, and sodium levels. Opt for products with lower added sugars, healthier fats (like monounsaturated and polyunsaturated fats), and higher fiber content.
- **Informed Dining**: When dining out, many restaurants now provide nutritional information for their menu items. Use this information to choose meals that align with your health goals, opting for dishes with balanced macronutrients and minimal added sugars or unhealthy fats.

Making these comparisons a habit will empower you to make smarter food choices, leading to a healthier overall diet.

Conclusion: Empowering Yourself with Knowledge

Understanding nutrition labels is about more than just numbers - it's about empowering yourself to take control of your diet and health. With this knowledge, you can confidently navigate the grocery store aisles, make informed choices, and align your food intake with your fitness and wellness goals.

As you continue your fitness journey, remember that every choice you make contributes to your overall health. By mastering the art of reading nutrition labels, you equip yourself with the tools to make decisions that nourish your body, support your goals, and enhance your quality of life. This knowledge is a powerful ally in your pursuit of a healthier, more balanced lifestyle.

CHAPTER 12:

SUPPLEMENTS - GOOD, BAD, AND THE USELESS

"Supplements are not a supplement for a balanced diet, but a complement to it"

– Anonymous

Supplements are a multi-billion dollar industry, with a staggering array of products lining the shelves of health stores and flooding online marketplaces. From protein powders and multivitamins to fat burners and detox teas, the sheer volume of options can be overwhelming. But amidst all the hype and marketing, how do you determine which supplements, if any, are truly beneficial? This chapter delves into the world of supplements, helping you understand when they might be necessary, which ones are backed by science, and how to make informed choices that support your health and fitness goals.

Do You Really Need Supplements?

The first question many people ask when they start a fitness journey or look to improve their health is whether they need to take supplements. The short answer is: it depends. While supplements can be helpful in certain situations, they are not a one-size-fits-all solution and should not replace a well-rounded diet rich in whole foods.

- **The Role of Whole Foods**: The foundation of any healthy diet should be whole, nutrient-dense foods. These include fruits, vegetables, lean proteins, whole grains, and healthy fats. Whole foods provide a complex array of vitamins, minerals, fiber, and phytonutrients that work synergistically to support overall health. For example, an orange offers more than just vitamin C; it also provides fiber, antioxidants, and a host of other beneficial compounds that supplements simply cannot replicate.

Think of supplements as the cherry on top of your nutritional sundae, not the entire dessert. They are meant to "supplement" your diet, not replace it. For most people, eating a balanced diet rich in a variety of foods will provide all the essential nutrients needed to support health and fitness.

- **When Supplements Might Be Necessary**: There are, however, situations where supplements can play a crucial role. If you have a specific nutrient deficiency, such as low iron levels (common in women), or vitamin D deficiency (prevalent in those who live in areas with limited sunlight), supplements can help fill the gap. Additionally, individuals with certain health conditions, such as osteoporosis, might benefit from supplements like calcium and vitamin D to support bone health.

Athletes and those engaged in intense physical training may also find that certain supplements, like protein powder or creatine, can aid in muscle recovery and performance. However, it's essential to approach supplements with caution and a clear understanding of your specific needs. Over-reliance on supplements can lead to imbalances and may not deliver the promised results if the rest of your diet is lacking.

Considerations: Before jumping into the supplement world, take stock of your overall diet and lifestyle. Are you regularly consuming a variety of fruits, vegetables, lean proteins, and healthy fats? Are you getting enough sleep, staying hydrated, and managing stress? These factors play a significant role in your overall health and should be the primary focus before considering supplements.

The Ones That Actually Work vs. Marketing Hype

The supplement industry is notorious for its marketing tactics, often promoting products with exaggerated claims that aren't backed by science. It's important to distinguish between supplements that have a solid foundation of research and those that are more about profit than health benefits.

- **Supplements with Solid Evidence**: Certain supplements have been extensively researched and shown to offer real benefits when used appropriately. These include:

    o **Protein Powder**: For those who struggle to meet their protein needs through food alone, especially athletes and those engaged in strength training, protein powder can be a convenient way to boost intake. Whey protein, in particular, is easily absorbed and has been shown to support muscle repair and growth when consumed after workouts.

- o **Omega-3 Fatty Acids**: Found in fish oil, omega-3 supplements are beneficial for heart health, reducing inflammation, and supporting brain function. If you don't regularly consume fatty fish like salmon, a high-quality omega-3 supplement can be a valuable addition to your diet.

- o **Vitamin D**: As mentioned earlier, vitamin D is crucial for bone health, immune function, and overall well-being. Many people, particularly those living in northern latitudes or with limited sun exposure, may benefit from supplementing with vitamin D, especially during the winter months.

- o **Creatine**: One of the most researched supplements for enhancing athletic performance, creatine has been shown to increase strength, improve high-intensity exercise performance, and support muscle mass gains. It's particularly popular among bodybuilders and athletes involved in power sports.

- **Supplements with Questionable Efficacy**: On the other end of the spectrum are supplements that promise miraculous results but lack scientific backing. These include:

  - o **Fat Burners**: Often marketed as the key to rapid weight loss, fat burners typically contain stimulants like caffeine and various herbs. While they might give a temporary energy boost, there's little evidence to support their effectiveness in long-term fat loss. Moreover, they can lead to jitteriness, anxiety, and even heart issues in some cases.

- o **Detox Teas**: Popularized by celebrities and influencers, detox teas claim to cleanse your body of toxins and promote weight loss. In reality, they often act as diuretics or laxatives, leading to temporary water weight loss and potentially harmful side effects like dehydration and electrolyte imbalances. Your liver and kidneys are already efficient at detoxifying your body - there's no need for these gimmicky products.

- o **Testosterone Boosters**: These supplements claim to increase testosterone levels and enhance muscle growth, particularly in men. However, most over-the-counter testosterone boosters have minimal impact on hormone levels and are unlikely to deliver the promised muscle gains. Unless prescribed by a healthcare professional for a specific deficiency, these products are often more hype than help.

Cautionary Note: When evaluating supplements, it's important to apply a healthy dose of scepticism. Look beyond the flashy marketing and ask critical questions: What evidence supports the claims made? Are the results from independent studies or company-sponsored research? Can the same benefits be achieved through diet and lifestyle changes alone? By approaching supplements with a critical eye, you can avoid wasting money on products that offer little more than placebo effects.

How to Choose the Right Supplements for You

Navigating the world of supplements can feel like a daunting task, but with the right approach, you can make informed decisions that align with your health and fitness goals. Here's a guide to help you choose the right supplements based on your needs, lifestyle, and goals.

- **Identify Your Needs**: Before adding any supplement to your routine, take a step back and assess what you're trying to achieve. Are you looking to build muscle, improve endurance, or address a specific nutrient deficiency? Understanding your goals will help you narrow down the supplements that might be beneficial.

    - **For General Health**: If you're simply looking to cover your nutritional bases, a high-quality multivitamin or omega-3 supplement might be sufficient, especially if your diet lacks certain nutrients.
    - **For Fitness Goals**: If you're focused on building muscle or improving recovery, protein powder, creatine, and branched-chain amino acids (BCAAs) might be worth considering.
    - **For Specific Deficiencies**: If you've been diagnosed with a deficiency, such as low iron or vitamin D, targeted supplements can help bring your levels back to normal. However, these should be taken under the guidance of a healthcare provider.

- **Read Labels Carefully**: Not all supplements are created equal, and the quality can vary significantly between brands. When choosing a supplement, read the labels carefully:

- ○ **Look for Reputable Brands**: Choose products from well-known, reputable companies that adhere to good manufacturing practices (GMP) and have third-party testing for quality and purity. Avoid brands that make exaggerated claims or rely on flashy marketing tactics.
- ○ **Check for Additives**: Some supplements contain unnecessary fillers, artificial colors, or sweeteners that can be avoided. Look for products with minimal additives and straightforward ingredient lists.
- ○ **Understand Dosages**: Pay attention to the dosage recommendations on the label and ensure they align with the latest scientific guidelines. Taking too much of a supplement can be as harmful as not taking enough.

— **Consult with Healthcare Providers**: Before starting any new supplement, especially if you have underlying health conditions or are taking other medications, it's crucial to consult with your healthcare provider. They can help determine whether the supplement is appropriate for you and whether it might interact with any medications you're currently taking.

Practical Tips: When you're considering a new supplement, do your research first. Look for studies published in peer-reviewed journals that support the claims made by the product. Check for any potential side effects and interactions with medications you may be taking. If possible, opt for supplements that have been third-party tested for purity and potency, as this adds an extra layer of assurance that you're getting what you pay for.

Conclusion: The Bottom Line on Supplements

Supplements can be a useful addition to your health and fitness regimen, but they should be approached with caution and care. The foundation of good nutrition lies in whole foods, and supplements should only be used to fill gaps or support specific goals. Always prioritize a balanced diet, and when considering supplements, choose those backed by science and aligned with your individual needs. Remember, no supplement can replace the benefits of a healthy diet and lifestyle, so let your food be your primary source of nutrients, and use supplements as a supportive tool on your wellness journey.

FITNESS IN ACTION: WORKOUTS AND PROGRESS TRACKING

CHAPTER 13:

CREATING A PERSONALIZED FITNESS PLAN

"There's no one-size-fits-all in fitness; it's personal"

– Anonymous

Crafting a personalized fitness plan is not just about picking exercises; it's about creating a sustainable and enjoyable routine that fits seamlessly into your life. This chapter will guide you through the process of setting realistic fitness goals, balancing fitness with other life commitments, and creating a flexible plan that adapts to your changing needs. The goal is to help you build a fitness routine that you can stick with for the long term, ensuring consistent progress and ongoing motivation.

How to Tailor Fitness to Your Lifestyle and Goals

When it comes to fitness, one of the biggest challenges is finding a routine that not only helps you reach your goals but also fits into your lifestyle. A personalized fitness plan is essential because what works for one person may not work for another. To create a plan that truly aligns with your needs, start by asking yourself a few key questions:

- **Identifying Your Goals**: The first step in creating a personalized fitness plan is identifying your goals. What do you want to achieve through your fitness routine? Your goals will guide every aspect of your plan, from the types of exercises you choose to the frequency and intensity of your workouts. Common fitness goals include:

  - **Weight Loss**: If your primary goal is weight loss, your plan might focus on a combination of cardiovascular exercises and strength training to help burn calories and build muscle mass, which in turn increases your metabolism.

  - **Muscle Building**: For those looking to build muscle, a plan centered around resistance training with progressive overload (gradually increasing weights) will be essential. Incorporating compound exercises like squats, deadlifts, and bench presses can help you maximize muscle growth.

  - **Improved Energy Levels**: If your goal is to feel more energetic, your plan might include a mix of moderate-intensity cardio and lighter strength training or yoga to boost your stamina and reduce fatigue.

  - **General Health and Wellness**: For those focused on overall health, a balanced mix of aerobic exercises, strength training, flexibility work, and activities like walking or cycling can help maintain a healthy weight, improve cardiovascular health, and enhance overall well-being.

Practical Application: Suppose your goal is to run a 10K race in six months. Your fitness plan should progressively build your endurance, starting with shorter runs and gradually increasing your distance and speed. You might also include strength training to improve your running efficiency and reduce the risk of injury. By aligning your fitness plan with your specific goal, you're more likely to stay motivated and see tangible progress.

- **Tailoring Your Plan to Fit Your Life**: The best fitness plan is one that you can actually stick to, and that means it needs to fit into your daily routine without feeling like a burden. Consider the following factors when tailoring your plan:

  - **Time Availability**: Assess your schedule to determine how much time you can realistically dedicate to fitness. If you have an hour each day, you might include a mix of cardio and strength training. If you're short on time, consider shorter, high-intensity workouts like HIIT that can be completed in 20-30 minutes but still deliver significant benefits.
  - **Preferred Time of Day**: Align your workouts with the time of day when you have the most energy and are least likely to encounter conflicts. If you're a morning person, a pre-work workout might be ideal. If you have more energy in the evening, an after-dinner session might work better.
  - **Location**: Decide whether you prefer working out at home, at a gym, or outdoors. If you enjoy being outside, incorporating activities like running, cycling, or hiking can make your fitness routine more enjoyable. If convenience is key, home workouts with minimal equipment might be the best option.

o **Practical Application**: Let's say you're a working parent with limited time in the mornings. A practical plan might involve a 30-minute workout right after the kids go to bed, focusing on a mix of bodyweight exercises and light cardio. This way, you can squeeze in your workout without disrupting your family routine.

Balancing Fitness with Work, Family, and Priorities

Life is busy, and finding time for fitness can often feel like an impossible task. However, with some strategic planning, it's entirely possible to balance fitness with work, family, and social obligations. The key is to integrate fitness into your life rather than seeing it as a separate, time-consuming task.

— **Scheduling Workouts Like Appointments**: One of the most effective ways to ensure consistency is to treat your workouts like any other important appointment. Schedule them into your calendar and prioritize them as you would a work meeting or a doctor's visit. By making your workouts non-negotiable, you're more likely to stick to your plan, even when life gets busy.

Practical Tip: If you're a professional with a demanding job, try scheduling your workouts first thing in the morning before the day's responsibilities pile up. This way, you've already accomplished something for yourself before the workday begins. Alternatively, if mornings are not an option, block out time during your lunch break for a quick gym session or a brisk walk.

- **Involving Your Family**: Fitness doesn't have to be a solo activity. Involving your family can make exercise more enjoyable and help you stay consistent. Whether it's going for a family bike ride, taking the dog for a walk together, or even playing a sport with your kids, turning fitness into a family affair can make it easier to incorporate into your daily life.

Practical Tip: On weekends, plan active outings with your family, such as hiking, swimming, or a visit to the park. Not only does this keep everyone moving, but it also fosters quality time together. If you have younger children, consider using a jogging stroller or baby carrier for your walks or runs, allowing you to stay active while caring for your little one.

- **Combining Social Activities with Exercise**: Social obligations don't have to derail your fitness goals. Instead of meeting friends for drinks or a meal, suggest an active outing like a walk, a hike, or even a group fitness class. This way, you can catch up with loved ones while staying active.

Practical Tip: If your social circle is not as fitness-oriented, you could still balance socializing and fitness by planning your workout before meeting up with friends. For instance, if you have a dinner planned, do a quick workout beforehand so you can enjoy the evening guilt-free. Another idea is to participate in charity walks or runs, where you can socialize while contributing to a good cause.

Creating a Flexible Plan for Long-Term Success

Flexibility is a crucial component of any successful fitness plan. Life is unpredictable, and there will be times when you need to adapt your routine. The key to long-term success is creating a plan that allows for adjustments without derailing your progress.

- **Adapting to Life's Changes**: Whether you're traveling, facing a busy period at work, or dealing with an injury, your fitness plan should be flexible enough to accommodate these changes. Rather than sticking rigidly to a plan that no longer fits, be willing to make adjustments as needed.

Practical Tip: If you're traveling for work or leisure, research hotels with gyms or nearby parks where you can get a workout in. If your usual routine involves an hour at the gym, but your schedule is suddenly packed, switch to shorter home workouts that require minimal equipment. Apps and online resources can be valuable tools for finding quick, effective workouts that can be done anywhere.

- **Listening to Your Body**: Pushing through fatigue or pain can lead to burnout or injury, which can set you back significantly. It's important to listen to your body and be willing to scale back when necessary. This might mean taking an extra rest day, opting for a lighter workout, or incorporating more recovery activities like stretching or yoga.

Practical Tip: Pay attention to how you feel during and after workouts. If you're consistently feeling exhausted or experiencing pain, it's a signal to reevaluate your plan. Perhaps you need to include more rest days, lower the intensity of your workouts, or focus more on recovery practices. Being attuned to your body's signals and adjusting your plan accordingly will help you avoid setbacks and maintain consistency.

- **Building in Flexibility**: Life doesn't always go according to plan, and neither does fitness. A rigid fitness plan might work in the short term, but for long-term success, it's essential to build in flexibility. This means being open to changing your routine when necessary and not beating yourself up if things don't go perfectly.

Practical Tip: Develop a "Plan B" for days when your regular workout isn't feasible. This might be a quick bodyweight circuit you can do at home, a brisk walk around your neighbourhood, or a yoga session to help you unwind. The goal is to keep moving, even if it's not your ideal workout. By having a flexible approach, you're more likely to stay consistent and avoid the all-or-nothing mentality that can lead to quitting.

Staying Motivated Over the Long Term: Keeping your fitness routine fresh and engaging is crucial for maintaining motivation. Periodically reassess your goals and consider trying new activities or setting new challenges for yourself. This could be anything from signing up for a race, trying a new fitness class, or setting a personal record in strength training. Keeping things varied and challenging helps prevent boredom and keeps you excited about your fitness journey.

Conclusion: Crafting a Fitness Plan That Lasts

Creating a personalized fitness plan is about more than just exercise; it's about integrating movement into your life in a way that is enjoyable, sustainable, and adaptable. By setting realistic goals, balancing fitness with other life commitments, and building in flexibility, you can create a fitness routine that supports your long-term health and wellness. Remember, the most effective fitness plan is one that fits seamlessly into your life, evolves with you, and keeps you motivated to stay active for the long haul.

CHAPTER 14

TRACKING PROGRESS WITHOUT LOSING YOUR MIND

"What gets measured gets managed"

– Peter Drucker

Tracking your fitness progress is an essential part of staying motivated and ensuring that you're moving toward your goals. However, it's easy to become overly focused on certain metrics, particularly the number on the scale, which can lead to frustration and discouragement. This chapter will explore various ways to measure success that go beyond the scale, the role of technology in tracking fitness, and how to maintain a healthy perspective while monitoring your progress.

— **Measuring Success Beyond the Scale**

The scale is often the go-to tool for tracking progress, especially when weight loss is a primary goal. However, it's important to recognize that the scale doesn't always tell the full story. Weight can fluctuate due to various factors, such as water retention, muscle gain, or even the time of day. Therefore, relying solely on the scale can be misleading and may not accurately reflect the positive changes happening in your body.

- **Body Composition**: One of the most effective ways to measure progress is by tracking changes in your body composition, specifically your body fat percentage. Unlike weight, body fat percentage provides a clearer picture of your overall health and fitness. For instance, if you're losing fat while gaining muscle, your weight might not change significantly, but your body composition will improve.

    - **How to Measure**: There are several ways to measure body fat percentage, ranging from calipers and bioelectrical impedance scales to more advanced methods like DEXA scans or hydrostatic weighing. While the more advanced methods are often more accurate, they can be expensive or less accessible. Calipers and bioelectrical impedance scales are convenient and can provide a reasonable estimate when used consistently.

- **Measurements and Clothing Fit**: Another practical way to track progress is by taking body measurements and noting how your clothes fit. This method can be particularly encouraging because it reflects changes that you can see and feel, even if the scale doesn't move.

    - **Key Measurements**: Focus on areas like your waist, hips, chest, arms, and thighs. Measure yourself at regular intervals - such as every two weeks - and record the results. Over time, you'll likely notice reductions in these measurements as you lose fat and build muscle.

- o **Clothing Fit**: Pay attention to how your clothes feel. Are your jeans getting looser around the waist? Does your shirt fit better in the shoulders? These are tangible signs of progress that often go unnoticed when focusing solely on the scale.

- **Strength and Endurance Gains**: Tracking improvements in strength and endurance is another excellent way to measure progress. As you continue your fitness journey, you'll likely find that you can lift heavier weights, complete more reps, or run longer distances than when you started.

  - o **Strength Tracking**: Keep a workout journal where you log the weights you lift and the number of sets and reps you complete. Over time, you should see these numbers increase, indicating that you're getting stronger.

  - o **Endurance Tracking**: Similarly, track your cardiovascular endurance by recording how long you can run, bike, swim, or perform other aerobic activities. As your endurance improves, you'll be able to sustain these activities for longer periods or at higher intensities.

  - o **Energy Levels and Overall Well-being**: One of the most significant yet often overlooked indicators of progress is how you feel. Increased energy levels, better sleep, reduced stress, and improved mood are all signs that your fitness routine is positively impacting your overall well-being.

- **Energy and Mood**: Keep a journal where you note your energy levels, mood, and overall feelings of well-being each day. As you become more consistent with your fitness routine, you'll likely notice improvements in these areas.

- **Sleep Quality**: Improved sleep is another key indicator of progress. If you're sleeping more soundly and waking up feeling refreshed, it's a sign that your body is adapting well to your fitness routine.

Perspective: Remember, success is multifaceted. The scale is just one tool, and it doesn't capture all the positive changes happening in your body. By broadening your definition of success, you can stay motivated and appreciate the full scope of your progress.

The Role of Technology in Tracking Fitness

In today's digital age, technology offers a variety of tools to help track and monitor your fitness progress. From wearable fitness trackers to smartphone apps and online platforms, these tools can provide valuable insights into your activity levels, sleep patterns, nutrition, and more. However, it's important to use technology as a supportive tool rather than becoming overly reliant on or obsessed with the data.

- **Benefits of Fitness Trackers and Apps**: Fitness trackers and apps can be powerful motivators. They provide real-time feedback on your activity levels, helping you stay on track with your goals. Here are some of the benefits of using these tools:

  o **Goal Setting**: Many apps and trackers allow you to set specific goals, such as a daily step count, calorie target, or workout frequency. These goals can help keep you focused and motivated.

- o **Activity Monitoring**: Trackers provide a detailed overview of your daily activity, including steps taken, distance travelled, and calories burned. This information can be useful for identifying patterns in your activity levels and making adjustments as needed.

- o **Sleep Tracking**: Some trackers monitor your sleep patterns, giving you insights into your sleep quality and duration. Improving sleep is crucial for recovery and overall well-being, and tracking it can help you identify areas for improvement.

- o **Nutrition Tracking**: Many apps allow you to log your meals and track your macronutrient intake. This can be especially helpful if you're following a specific diet plan or trying to ensure you're getting enough protein, carbs, and fats.

- **Form Factors and Capabilities**: Fitness tracking devices come in various forms, each with its own set of features and capabilities. Understanding these differences can help you choose the right tool for your needs:

  - o **Watches**: Fitness watches are the most popular form factor and typically offer a wide range of features, including heart rate monitoring, GPS tracking, step counting, and notifications. They are suitable for users who want a comprehensive overview of their fitness and daily activities.

  - o **Bracelets**: Fitness bracelets are often more streamlined and may focus on essential metrics like steps, calories, and sleep. They are ideal for users who prefer a simpler, less obtrusive device.

- o **Rings**: Fitness rings are discreet and focus primarily on sleep and recovery metrics. They are a good choice for users who want to track their health without wearing a larger device.
- o **Chest Straps**: Chest straps provide highly accurate heart rate monitoring and are often used by serious athletes during high-intensity training. They are less common for everyday use but are valuable for those who need precise data.
- o **Smartphone Apps**: Many users opt for smartphone apps that can track activities using the phone's built-in sensors. These apps often include features for tracking workouts, nutrition, and overall health.

- **Accuracy and Features**: The accuracy of fitness trackers can vary depending on the type of device and the metric being measured. For example:

- o **Heart Rate Monitoring**: Watches and chest straps generally offer accurate heart rate data, with chest straps being the most precise. However, accuracy can decrease during activities involving wrist movement, such as weightlifting.
- o **GPS Tracking**: Watches with built-in GPS are highly accurate for tracking outdoor activities like running or cycling. Bracelets and rings typically do not include GPS, making them less suitable for precise distance tracking.
- o **Sleep Tracking**: Rings and bracelets tend to excel in sleep tracking, offering detailed insights into sleep stages and quality. Watches also provide sleep data but may be less comfortable to wear overnight.

Popular Features:

- **ECG Monitoring**: Some advanced trackers include electrocardiogram (ECG) capabilities, allowing users to monitor heart rhythm and detect potential abnormalities.
- **Oxygen Saturation (SpO2)**: Many devices now offer SpO2 monitoring, which measures blood oxygen levels and can be useful for detecting sleep apnea or monitoring respiratory health.
- **Stress and Recovery Metrics**: Some trackers provide insights into stress levels and recovery, using metrics like heart rate variability (HRV) to gauge overall well-being.
- **Integration with Other Apps**: Many trackers integrate with third-party apps for nutrition, meditation, or workout programs, offering a holistic approach to health.

Practical Use: To make the most of your fitness tracker, start by setting realistic goals that align with your fitness plan. Use the data to guide your decisions but remember to listen to your body. If your tracker shows you haven't hit your step goal for the day but you're feeling exhausted, it's okay to rest. The data is there to inform you, not dictate your every move.

- **Drawbacks and Potential Pitfalls**: While technology can be incredibly useful, there are potential drawbacks to be aware of. It's easy to become overly focused on numbers, which can lead to stress, anxiety, or unhealthy behaviours.
  - **Data Overload**: Constantly monitoring your stats can lead to information overload. Instead of

motivating you, it can become overwhelming, leading to burnout or discouragement if you don't meet your targets.

- **Over-Reliance on Technology**: While trackers provide valuable data, they can't measure everything. For example, they might not accurately capture the intensity of strength training workouts or the benefits of yoga and stretching. Relying too much on technology can cause you to lose sight of the broader picture of your fitness and well-being.

- **Obsessive Behaviour**: Becoming fixated on numbers - whether it's steps, calories, or heart rate - can lead to obsessive behaviour. It's important to use the data as a guide rather than allowing it to control your life. Remember that fitness is about more than just hitting specific targets; it's about feeling good, being healthy, and enjoying the process.

Balanced Approach: To avoid these pitfalls, set boundaries for your use of technology. For example, you might choose to check your stats at the end of the day rather than constantly throughout. Or, you might decide to have one day a week where you don't use your tracker at all, focusing instead on how you feel. The key is to use technology as a tool to enhance your fitness journey, not as something that creates additional stress.

Conclusion: Progress Is More Than Numbers

Tracking your fitness progress is crucial for staying motivated and on course, but it's essential to approach it with a balanced mindset. The scale is just one of many tools you can use to measure success, and it's not always the most accurate reflection of your progress. By focusing on a variety of indicators - such as body composition, strength, endurance, and overall well-being - you can get a more comprehensive view of your fitness journey.

Technology can be a valuable ally in tracking your progress, but it's important to use it wisely. Avoid becoming overly reliant on numbers and data, and remember to listen to your body. Celebrate small victories, maintain a long-term perspective, and find joy in the process. By doing so, you'll stay motivated, avoid burnout, and continue making progress without losing your mind along the way. Fitness is a marathon, not a sprint, and the journey is just as important as the destination.

THE MINDSET

CHAPTER 15

MOTIVATION - KEEPING THE FIRE BURNING

"Your motivation is your compass, it guides you
when the path gets tough"

– Anonymous

Motivation is the engine that drives your fitness journey, but like any engine, it needs fuel. Staying motivated is often the hardest part of maintaining a healthy lifestyle, especially when life gets busy or progress seems slow. This chapter will help you identify your deeper motivations, offer strategies for staying motivated on tough days, and explore the power of accountability and community support in keeping your fire burning.

Finding Your "Why"

To sustain long-term motivation, it's crucial to connect with a deeper purpose - your "why." While it's common to start a fitness journey with goals related to physical appearance, such as losing weight or building muscle, these surface-level goals often aren't enough to keep you going when the initial excitement wears off.

To stay committed, you need to dig deeper and find a purpose that resonates on a personal level.

— **Identifying Deeper Motivations**: Ask yourself why you really want to get fit. What are the underlying reasons beyond the desire to look good? Is it to improve your health and increase your lifespan? To have more energy to play with your kids or grandkids? To reduce stress and improve your mental health? Perhaps it's to build confidence, feel more comfortable in your own skin, or regain control over your body after a period of inactivity or illness.

  o **Reflective Exercise**: Take a moment to write down your reasons for wanting to improve your fitness. Be honest with yourself and dig deep to uncover motivations that are meaningful and personal to you. For example, instead of saying, "I want to lose weight," you might write, "I want to lose weight so I can manage my blood pressure and be there for my family in the long run."

  o **Visualizing Your "Why"**: Visualization can be a powerful tool for keeping your motivation alive. Close your eyes and imagine what your life will look like once you've achieved your fitness goals. How will you feel? How will your relationships and daily activities improve? Creating a mental picture of your success can help keep you motivated, especially when challenges arise.

— **Keeping Your "Why" Front and Center**: Once you've identified your deeper motivations, it's important to keep them front and center in your daily life. This could mean writing them down and placing them somewhere visible, like on your bathroom mirror, or setting reminders on your phone. By regularly reminding yourself of your "why," you reinforce your commitment and keep your goals aligned with your deeper purpose.

How to Stay Motivated on Tough Days

Even the most motivated individuals have days when they struggle to find the energy or desire to work out. The key to staying on track during these times is to have a strategy in place for those tough days. By setting small, achievable goals, rewarding progress, and mixing up your routines, you can keep your motivation alive even when it feels like it's slipping away.

— **Setting Small, Achievable Goals**: Large, long-term goals can sometimes feel overwhelming, especially when progress is slow. Breaking down these big goals into smaller, more manageable steps can make the journey feel less daunting and give you frequent opportunities to celebrate success.

  o **Incremental Progress**: For example, if your goal is to run a marathon, start by setting a goal to run a 5K, then a 10K, and so on. Each time you reach one of these smaller milestones, you'll feel a sense of accomplishment that fuels your motivation to keep going.

  o **Daily and Weekly Goals**: In addition to long-term goals, set daily or weekly goals that are easy to achieve. This could be as simple as committing to a 10-minute walk each day or trying a new workout once a week. These small victories can build momentum and help you stay consistent.

- **Rewarding Progress**: Positive reinforcement is a powerful motivator. Rewarding yourself for hitting milestones, no matter how small, can help keep your motivation high. Rewards don't have to be extravagant - sometimes, a little treat or a new piece of workout gear is enough to keep you going.

  - **Types of Rewards**: Consider non-food rewards that support your fitness journey. For example, treat yourself to a relaxing massage after completing a month of consistent workouts, buy a new workout outfit, or take a day trip to a favorite hiking spot. These rewards not only celebrate your achievements but also reinforce the healthy habits you're building.

  - **Celebrating Small Victories**: Don't wait until you reach your ultimate goal to celebrate. Each step forward is worth recognizing. Celebrate the small victories - whether it's lifting heavier weights, increasing your running distance, or simply sticking to your workout plan for the week. These celebrations help you stay motivated by acknowledging your progress.

- **Mixing Up Routines to Keep Things Fresh**: One of the biggest motivation killers is monotony. Doing the same workouts day in and day out can lead to boredom and burnout. Keeping your routine fresh and engaging is key to maintaining long-term motivation.

  - **Variety in Workouts**: Try incorporating different types of exercise into your routine. If you usually run, add strength training, yoga, or cycling to the mix. If you're into weightlifting, consider adding some cardio or flexibility exercises. The change will not only keep things interesting but also help prevent plateaus by challenging your body in new ways.

- o **Trying New Activities**: Don't be afraid to step out of your comfort zone and try something new. Take a dance class, try rock climbing, or join a group fitness class you've never done before. New activities can reignite your excitement for fitness and introduce you to new skills and challenges.

— **Accountability Partners and Fitness Communities**

Staying motivated can be easier when you're not doing it alone. Having an accountability partner or being part of a fitness community can provide the support, encouragement, and friendly competition needed to keep you on track. Whether it's a workout buddy, a family member, or an online group, these relationships can play a crucial role in maintaining your motivation.

- — **The Power of Accountability**: Knowing that someone else is counting on you can be a powerful motivator. When you have an accountability partner, you're less likely to skip a workout or stray from your goals because you don't want to let them down.

- o **Finding an Accountability Partner**: Look for someone who shares similar goals or interests. This could be a friend, family member, or coworker who also wants to stay fit. Set up regular workout dates, check-ins, or even friendly challenges to keep each other motivated.

- o **Benefits of Accountability**: Accountability partners can provide encouragement on tough days, celebrate your successes with you, and help you stay committed to your goals. They also offer a sense of camaraderie, making the fitness journey feel less solitary.

— **Joining a Fitness Community**: Being part of a fitness community, whether in person or online, can provide an additional layer of support. These communities offer a space to share experiences, ask for advice, and find inspiration from others who are on similar journeys.

- o **Types of Communities**: Fitness communities come in many forms, from local running clubs and gym classes to online forums and social media groups. Find a community that aligns with your interests and goals. For example, if you're into yoga, join a local studio or an online yoga community where you can connect with like-minded individuals.

- o **Engaging with Your Community**: Don't just join a community - actively engage with it. Participate in discussions, attend events, and offer support to others. The more involved you are, the more benefits you'll gain from the community. Sharing your journey and hearing about others' experiences can be incredibly motivating.

Conclusion: Fuel the Fire: Staying Motivated for the Long Haul

Motivation is the spark that ignites your fitness journey, but sustaining it requires commitment, self-awareness, and the right support system. By identifying your deeper "why," embracing small wins, and surrounding yourself with a community that encourages growth, you create a foundation for lasting success. Some days will be harder than others, but remember that consistency, not perfection, is the key to progress. When motivation wanes, rely on discipline and the habits you've built to keep moving forward. Ultimately, the journey to fitness is not just about physical transformation but about discovering your inner strength, resilience, and the joy of becoming the best version of yourself.

CHAPTER 16

THE POWER OF HABITS

> "We are what we repeatedly do. Excellence,
> then, is not an act, but a habit"

– Aristotle

While motivation gets you started, habits are what keep you going. Building and sticking to healthy routines is key to long-term success. In this chapter, you'll learn about the science of habit formation, the power of small changes, and why consistency beats perfection every time.

Building and Sticking to Healthy Routines

Creating new habits can feel daunting, but understanding how habits are formed can make the process easier. Habits are behaviours that become automatic over time through repetition. The good news is that once a habit is established, it requires less mental effort to maintain, making it easier to stay consistent.

- **The Science of Habit Formation**: Habits are formed through a loop that involves a cue, a routine, and a reward. The cue triggers the behaviour, the routine is the behaviour itself, and the reward reinforces the behaviour, making you more likely to repeat it in the future.

- o **Cue**: The cue can be anything that prompts you to start your routine. For example, setting out your workout clothes the night before can serve as a cue to exercise in the morning.
- o **Routine**: The routine is the habit you want to establish, such as going for a run, drinking water first thing in the morning, or preparing a healthy breakfast.
- o **Reward**: The reward is what you get out of completing the routine. It could be the endorphin rush after a workout, the satisfaction of ticking off a task, or simply feeling energized for the day. Identifying a reward that's meaningful to you will help reinforce the habit.

Practical Example: If your goal is to build a habit of morning exercise, your cue might be laying out your workout clothes before bed. The routine is the workout itself, and the reward could be a post-workout smoothie or the satisfaction of starting your day on a positive note. Over time, this loop becomes ingrained, making it easier to stick to your routine.

- — **Starting Small and Building Success**: One of the biggest mistakes people make when trying to establish new habits is trying to change too much too quickly. Starting small allows you to build success gradually, making it more likely that your new habits will stick.

  - o **Micro-Habits**: Micro-habits are small, easy-to-do behaviours that serve as the building blocks for larger changes. For example, if your goal is to eat healthier, start by adding one serving of vegetables to your dinner each night. Once that habit is established, you can build on it by making more healthy swaps in your diet.

o **Gradual Progression**: As you become consistent with your micro-habits, gradually increase the challenge. For instance, if you've started with a 5-minute morning stretch routine, add 5 more minutes each week until you're doing a full workout. This approach prevents burnout and makes the process of building new habits feel manageable.

Practical Example: If you're new to exercise, start with just 10 minutes a day. Once you've consistently done this for a few weeks, increase the duration or intensity. By the time you reach your full workout length, the habit will already be firmly established.

How Small Changes Make a Big Difference

The idea that small changes can lead to significant results is a powerful concept. When you make small, consistent changes to your habits, these changes compound over time, leading to lasting improvements in your health and fitness.

— **The Power of Incremental Change**: Incremental changes may seem insignificant at first, but they add up over time. For example, swapping a sugary snack for a piece of fruit each day might not seem like much, but over the course of a year, that simple change could lead to weight loss and improved health.

- o **Compounding Effects**: Think of small changes as investments in your health. Just as financial investments grow over time due to compounding interest, small, positive changes in your habits can lead to significant improvements in your fitness and well-being.
- o **Avoiding Overwhelm**: Small changes are also easier to stick with than drastic overhauls. By focusing on one change at a time, you avoid feeling overwhelmed and are more likely to succeed in the long term.

Practical Example: If your goal is to increase your daily activity, start by taking the stairs instead of the elevator, parking farther from the store entrance, or going for a short walk after dinner. These small actions might seem minor, but over time, they can significantly boost your daily activity levels and improve your health.

- — **The Ripple Effect**: Often, making one positive change can lead to others. For example, starting a morning exercise routine might lead to healthier eating habits throughout the day because you don't want to undo the good work you've done. This ripple effect can create a positive feedback loop that makes it easier to adopt and maintain healthy habits.

  - o **Building Momentum**: As you make small changes and see positive results, you'll build momentum that makes it easier to continue improving. Each success reinforces your commitment and motivates you to keep going.

- o **Practical Example**: If you start by improving your hydration habits - drinking a glass of water before each meal - you might find that you naturally start making healthier food choices because you're more mindful of your overall well-being. This small change can lead to better digestion, increased energy levels, and even improved skin health, creating a ripple effect of positive outcomes.

The Importance of Consistency Over Perfection

In the pursuit of fitness goals, it's easy to fall into the trap of seeking perfection. However, striving for perfection can lead to frustration, burnout, and ultimately, failure. The key to long-term success is consistency, not perfection.

- **Showing Up Regularly**: Consistency means showing up and doing the work regularly, even when you don't feel like it or when circumstances aren't ideal. It's about making fitness a non-negotiable part of your life, rather than something you do only when conditions are perfect.

  - o **The 80/20 Rule**: The 80/20 rule, also known as the Pareto Principle, can be applied to fitness. It suggests that 80% of your results come from 20% of your efforts. This means that you don't have to be perfect all the time to see progress - what matters most is consistently doing the things that have the biggest impact on your goals.

  - o **Avoiding All-Or-Nothing Thinking**: Perfectionism often leads to an all-or-nothing mindset, where you either do something perfectly or not at all. This can be a recipe for failure, as it sets you up to quit when you inevitably fall short. Instead, focus on progress over perfection and recognize that small, consistent efforts add up over time.

Practical Example: If you miss a workout or have an indulgent meal, don't beat yourself up or throw in the towel. Instead, get back on track the next day and keep moving forward. One slip-up doesn't erase all your progress - what matters is how you respond and your ability to maintain consistency over the long term.

- **Forgiving Yourself for Slip-Ups**: Everyone has setbacks, whether it's missing a few workouts, indulging in unhealthy foods, or feeling unmotivated. The key is to forgive yourself for these slip-ups and move on. Holding onto guilt or frustration only makes it harder to get back on track.

  - **Learning from Setbacks**: Instead of seeing slip-ups as failures, view them as learning opportunities. Ask yourself what led to the setback and how you can avoid similar situations in the future. By reflecting on your experiences, you can develop strategies to overcome obstacles and stay consistent.
  - **Focusing on the Long-Term**: Remember that fitness is a marathon, not a sprint. One bad day or week doesn't define your journey. What matters most is the overall trend - are you making progress over time? Keep your focus on the long-term goal and don't let temporary setbacks derail your efforts.

Practical Example: If you miss a week of workouts due to a busy schedule or illness, don't get discouraged. Instead, ease back into your routine and remind yourself of your long-term goals. Consistency is about making fitness a part of your lifestyle, not about being perfect every single day.

- **Celebrating Consistency**: Celebrate your consistency just as you would any other achievement. Recognize that showing up regularly, even when it's tough, is a victory in itself. By celebrating your consistency, you reinforce the habit and motivate yourself to keep going.

Practical Example: If you've been consistent with your workouts for a month, treat yourself to something that supports your fitness journey, like a new pair of running shoes or a massage. These rewards reinforce the importance of consistency and help you stay committed to your goals.

Conclusion: The Mindset for Long-Term Success

Staying motivated, building healthy habits, and embracing consistency are all key elements of a successful fitness journey. By finding your deeper "why," staying motivated on tough days, and leaning on accountability and community, you can keep the fire burning even when the going gets tough. Remember, it's the small, consistent actions that lead to big changes over time. Embrace the process, celebrate your progress, and stay committed to the long-term journey. With the right mindset, there's nothing you can't achieve.

06

DEBUNKING THE MYTHS & EMBRACING THE JOURNEY

CHAPTER 17

MYTHBUSTERS

"Don't let myths guide your life; seek the truth"

– Anonymous

Introduction to Myths in Fitness and Nutrition

In today's world, we are constantly bombarded with information - much of it from social media, where anyone with a platform can share their opinions on fitness and nutrition. Unfortunately, this has led to a proliferation of myths and misconceptions that can be harmful, leading to confusion, wasted time, and even health risks. In this chapter, we'll dive deep into some of the most pervasive myths in fitness and nutrition, separating the science from the snake oil so you can make informed decisions about your health.

"We live in the age of information - and misinformation. With every scroll through your social media feed, you're bombarded with the latest 'miracle diet' or 'must-try workout.' But how much of it is actually true? Unfortunately, a lot of what you see is more fiction than fact. In this chapter, we're going to bust some of the most common myths in fitness and nutrition so you can separate the science from the snake oil."

Myth 1: "Carbs Are the Enemy"

Carbohydrates have been demonized in recent years, especially with the rise of low-carb diets like keto and Atkins. The myth that carbs are inherently bad and should be avoided for weight loss has taken hold, leading many to fear this essential macronutrient. However, the reality is that carbohydrates are your body's primary source of energy, especially for those who are active.

Carbs are not the enemy - your body needs them to function optimally. The key is to choose the right types of carbohydrates. Complex carbs, found in whole grains, fruits, and vegetables, provide sustained energy and are packed with nutrients. They differ significantly from simple carbs, which are often refined and stripped of their nutritional value. Simple carbs, like those found in sugary snacks, can lead to spikes and crashes in blood sugar levels.

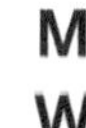

Myth 2: "Do Detoxes and Cleanses to Lose Weight"

Detoxes and cleanses are often marketed as quick fixes for weight loss or as a way to "reset" your body. But the idea that your body needs help to detoxify is a myth. Your body already has a highly effective detoxification system in place - your liver and kidneys are working 24/7 to filter out toxins and waste.

Detox diets can be harmful, often involving extreme calorie restrictions or consuming only liquids, which can lead to nutrient deficiencies, muscle loss, and a slowed metabolism. Instead of resorting to these extreme measures, focus on a balanced diet that supports your body's natural processes.

Myth 3: "Lifting Weights Will Make You Bulky"

Many people, particularly women, shy away from lifting weights for fear of becoming bulky. This myth persists despite the fact that building significant muscle mass requires a specific combination of factors, including genetics, diet, and an intense training regimen.

The truth is, lifting weights helps you build lean muscle, which in turn increases your metabolism and improves your overall strength and fitness. Strength training is crucial for maintaining muscle mass as you age, supporting bone density, and enhancing functional strength. It's not about turning into the Hulk; it's about building a strong, healthy body.

Myth 4: "You Can Spot-Reduce Fat"

The idea of spot-reducing fat - losing fat in specific areas by targeting them with exercise - is a persistent myth. Whether it's doing crunches to lose belly fat or leg lifts to slim your thighs, the truth is that fat loss doesn't work this way.

Fat loss occurs across the entire body and is driven by creating a calorie deficit, where you burn more calories than you consume. While targeted exercises can strengthen and tone specific muscles, they won't reduce fat in those areas alone. To lose fat, focus on a combination of cardiovascular exercise, strength training, and a balanced diet.

Myth 5: "More Exercise is Always Better"

There's a common misconception that more exercise automatically leads to better results. While it's important to stay active, overtraining can lead to burnout, injury, and diminished returns.

Rest and recovery are just as important as the exercise itself. Your muscles need time to repair and grow stronger after workouts. Overtraining can lead to fatigue, decreased performance, and even an increased risk of illness. A balanced fitness routine includes a mix of exercise, rest, and recovery to keep your body performing at its best.

Myth 6: "Fad Diets Are the Key to Quick Weight Loss"

Fad diets often promise quick results with little effort - lose 10 pounds in a week! But these diets are rarely sustainable and often lead to yo-yo dieting, where you lose weight only to gain it back (and sometimes more) once the diet ends.

Fad diets typically involve extreme calorie restrictions, eliminating entire food groups, or relying on single-food diets, all of which can be harmful to your physical and mental health. These diets can lead to nutrient deficiencies, muscle loss, and a slowed metabolism. Instead, focus on balanced, sustainable eating habits that you can maintain for the long term. Real, lasting change comes from consistency, not quick fixes.

Myth 7: "You Must Avoid All Fat to Stay Healthy"

For years, fat was the villain in the world of nutrition, blamed for everything from heart disease to obesity. But not all fats are created equal. The key is distinguishing between unhealthy fats, like trans fats and excessive saturated fats, and healthy fats, like monounsaturated and polyunsaturated fats.

Healthy fats are essential for your body's function - they support brain health, hormone production, and nutrient absorption. Sources of healthy fats include avocados, nuts, seeds, and olive oil. Rather than avoiding fat altogether, focus on incorporating these healthy fats into your diet in moderation.

Myth 8: "Social Media Influencers Know Best"

Scrolling through social media can feel like navigating a minefield of misinformation, especially when it comes to fitness and nutrition. Influencers with perfect abs and glowing skin might seem like they have all the answers, but many are promoting trends rather than science-based advice.

These influencers often lack the credentials or expertise to provide sound health advice, yet their visually appealing content can easily mislead followers. The problem with following such advice is that it can lead to unrealistic expectations, frustration, and even harm. For example, you might be tempted to try a restrictive diet that promises quick results but ends up damaging your metabolism or mental health. Or you might follow a workout routine designed for someone with a different fitness level, leading to injury.

When it comes to your health, it's crucial to seek advice from qualified professionals - dietitians, nutritionists, and certified trainers - who can provide guidance based on evidence, not trends. Critically evaluate the information you consume online and remember that popularity doesn't equate to accuracy.

 Myth 9: "Healthy Food is Always Expensive"

There's a widespread belief that eating healthy is expensive and out of reach for many people. While it's true that some health foods can be pricey, there are plenty of affordable, nutritious options available.

Whole foods like beans, lentils, oats, vegetables, and seasonal fruits are not only budget-friendly but also packed with nutrients. Planning your meals, buying in bulk, and cooking at home can significantly reduce the cost of eating healthily. You don't need to buy expensive superfoods or organic everything to eat well; focus on simple, whole foods that fit your budget.

Final Thoughts on Myths

As you navigate your journey towards better health and fitness, it's essential to be aware of the myths and misinformation that can lead you astray. These myths can create unnecessary stress, waste your time and money, and even jeopardize your health. By approaching fitness and nutrition with a critical eye and prioritizing evidence-based practices, you can build a sustainable, healthy lifestyle that works for you.

Your health is too important to be left to myths and misinformation. Take the time to educate yourself, seek advice from qualified professionals, and prioritize practices that are grounded in science. When you do, you'll find that the path to health and wellness is not about quick fixes or extreme measures but about making informed choices that support your well-being every day.

CHAPTER 18

THE JOURNEY CONTINUES

"What you seek is seeking you"

– Rumi

As you come to the end of this book, it's important to reflect on the idea that fitness is not just a goal or a destination but a continuous journey. This journey, much like life itself, is filled with growth, learning, adaptation, and transformation. As you step into your 40s and beyond, this journey takes on new significance. It becomes an opportunity to redefine what fitness means to you, explore new horizons, and deepen your commitment to a healthy and fulfilling life.

Embracing Fitness as a Lifelong Journey

Throughout this book, we've delved into the foundational elements of a healthy lifestyle: nutrition, exercise, mindset, and habits. Each chapter has created a comprehensive approach to fitness that is both sustainable and adaptable. However, fitness is not about reaching a single point of success. It's about embracing the journey and recognizing that your health and well-being are ever-evolving.

In your 40s, 50s, and beyond, you enter a phase rich with potential. You have the wisdom of experience, resilience from overcoming challenges, and clarity about what truly matters. This is a time to harness these strengths and elevate your fitness journey.

Consider how your approach to fitness has evolved. In your younger days, it might have been driven by aesthetics or performance. Now, fitness is about how you feel, move, and live. It's about activities that bring joy, enhance your quality of life, and keep you active and healthy into later years. Whether maintaining mobility, reducing stress, or feeling strong, the focus shifts to goals that align with your current needs and desires.

For instance, if high-intensity workouts now strain your joints, explore gentler options like swimming, yoga, or Pilates. These activities support your physical health and offer mental and emotional benefits, keeping you balanced and centered.

Reflect on the lessons you've learned in this book: understanding calories, finding your calorie sweet spot, realizing the importance of strength training, and embracing movement beyond the gym. These tools have set you up for a sustainable, active lifestyle. Now, it's up to you to continue applying these lessons.

How to Stay Flexible and Adapt as Your Body Changes

A lifelong fitness journey requires adaptability. As you age, your body changes, presenting both challenges and opportunities.

Instead of resisting these changes, embrace them as part of your evolution. Flexibility in your routine and mindset is key.

Recognizing and Embracing Change

Physical abilities shift with age. Recovery may take longer, or some exercises may become uncomfortable. These changes don't mean you must give up fitness; they simply require adjustments.

Adaptation is Strength

Just as you've adapted to challenges in other areas of life, you can modify your fitness routine to suit your current needs. If high-impact exercises feel taxing, try low-impact options like cycling or water aerobics. These are gentle on joints yet provide excellent cardiovascular benefits.

Focus on Mobility and Flexibility

Maintaining mobility and flexibility becomes increasingly important. Incorporating practices like yoga, Pilates, or tai chi helps sustain range of motion, reduces injury risk, and improves overall quality of life. These activities also promote mindfulness and relaxation, enhancing both physical and mental health.

For example, if running now strains your knees, consider transitioning to cycling or hiking. These activities offer cardiovascular benefits while reducing joint impact.

Listening to Your Body's Signals

Your body constantly communicates its needs. Tuning into these signals and responding appropriately is crucial for avoiding injury and staying healthy.

- **Prioritizing Recovery**: Recovery becomes essential as you age. Incorporate rest days, prioritize sleep, and use practices like stretching or massage therapy to support recovery.
- **Adjusting Expectations**: Performance evolves with age. Focus on what you can do rather than what you used to do. Celebrate your body's ability to adapt and stay strong.

For instance, if heavy strength training no longer feels good on your joints, adjust by using lighter weights, resistance bands, or bodyweight exercises. This approach allows you to build strength safely.

The Journey is the Destination

The most important aspect of your fitness journey is the commitment to your health and well-being. Fitness goes beyond physical strength; it encompasses mental resilience, emotional balance, and determination to live your best life.

Embrace Your Capabilities at Any Age

You can achieve fitness goals at any age. Whether you're 40, 50, or beyond, you have the power to improve your health and enhance your quality of life. Approach your journey with growth, resilience, and optimism.

A Shift in Mindset

Fitness is not just about appearance or performance. It's about feeling good in your body, moving through life with energy, and approaching each day with enthusiasm. This mindset shift sustains your fitness journey over the long term.

Enjoy the Process

Successful fitness journeys come from finding joy in the process. Fitness should be something you look forward to. Whether it's a yoga session's calm focus or the simple pleasure of moving your body, find activities that bring happiness.

For example, starting a new activity like dance or tennis might initially focus on skill mastery. Over time, you'll find the true joy lies in participating and enjoying the process rather than perfecting it.

Stay Positive and Resilient

Fitness, like life, has ups and downs. There will be days when motivation wanes or challenges arise. In these moments, stay positive and resilient.

- **Forgive Yourself**: If you miss a workout or indulge in an unhealthy meal, don't let it derail your progress. Fitness is a long-term commitment.
- **Keep the Big Picture in Mind**: Temporary setbacks don't define your journey. Focus on your overall progress and commitment to staying active and healthy.

For instance, after a tough week, plan a workout or prepare healthy meals to get back on track. Resilience and a positive outlook help you bounce back stronger.

Final Thoughts: The Journey Is Yours to Continue

Your fitness journey is uniquely yours, and it will continue to evolve. Each chapter of this book has equipped you with tools and knowledge for a healthy, active lifestyle that adapts to your needs. Now, it's up to you to apply these lessons.

Your journey is far from over; it's just beginning. Embrace each phase of life with enthusiasm and commitment to your well-being. Keep moving, learning, and exploring what fitness means to you. The possibilities are endless, and the best is yet to come.

WHY THIS BOOK MATTERS TO ALL AGES

"The essence of health and vitality transcends age; it's a pursuit for everyone, at any stage of life"

– Anonymous

Fitness is a journey, not a destination. Whether you're in your 20s, 30s, 50s, or beyond, the principles of health, fitness, and well-being that we explore together are universally applicable and beneficial.

Throughout this book, we've delved into key areas like strength training, nutrition, sleep, and the importance of movement beyond the gym. Each of these areas holds relevance for adults at any stage of life. This chapter will explore how the advice, tips, and strategies discussed in previous chapters are just as valuable for anyone looking to improve their health, regardless of their starting point.

Universal Principles of Fitness

At the core of a healthy lifestyle are a few key principles that apply to everyone, regardless of age. Strength training, balanced nutrition, proper hydration, and quality sleep are the foundation of good health. While our needs and goals may shift as we age, these elements remain consistent, forming the bedrock of any effective fitness plan.

Strength Training: As discussed in Chapter 3, *Why Strength Training is Non-Negotiable After 40,* strength training is critical not just for maintaining muscle mass as we age, but for building it at any stage of life. Whether you're aiming to enhance your performance in your 20s or preserve your independence in your 60s, strength training is a must. It supports bone density, joint stability, and functional strength, making it an essential component of overall health.

Balanced Nutrition: The importance of nutrition has been emphasized throughout this book, especially in Part 3, *Nutrition – Eating Smart, Not Less.* No matter your age, balanced nutrition is crucial. Younger adults might focus on fuelling their bodies for growth and energy, while older adults need to ensure they're consuming nutrient-dense foods that support metabolic health, muscle retention, and overall well-being.

Hydration: In Chapter 5, *Section: Why Staying Hydrated is Critical, Especially Now,* we explored how vital water is for every bodily function - from regulating temperature to aiding digestion. Staying hydrated is crucial for maintaining health at any age. It supports physical performance, cognitive function, and overall vitality.

Sleep: As highlighted in Chapter 4, *Sleep – Your Secret Weapon,* sleep is the body's natural recovery mechanism. Quality sleep is essential for muscle recovery, mental clarity, and emotional well-being, whether you're a busy professional in your 30s or enjoying retirement in your 70s. Prioritizing sleep is key to living a healthy, balanced life.

These principles form the foundation of fitness, and they are just as relevant at 25 as they are at 45 or 65. While the specific ways we apply these principles may change over time, their importance remains unchanged.

Long-Term Benefits of Early Adoption

Adopting these universal principles early in life sets the stage for healthier aging. The habits you establish in your 20s or 30s - whether it's regular strength training, balanced eating, staying hydrated, or prioritizing sleep - will pay dividends as you grow older.

As discussed in Chapter 15, *Motivation – Keeping the Fire Burning,* it's about finding your personal motivation and starting where you are. Whether you're beginning your fitness journey in your 20s, 30s, 40s, 50s, or beyond, integrating these practices into your daily life can lead to significant improvements in your health and quality of life.

Adapting Strategies Across Ages

The beauty of fitness is that it can be tailored to meet you where you are in life. The strategies outlined in this book can be customized to suit the unique needs and goals of different age groups.

For those in their 20s and 30s, the focus might be on building endurance and exploring a variety of physical activities. This is the time to experiment, challenge yourself, and lay down a solid fitness foundation, as discussed in Chapter 3, *Section, Easy-to-Follow Beginner's Guide to Strength Training.* Strength training, high-intensity workouts, and adventurous outdoor activities can help build the stamina and resilience that will serve you well in the decades to come.

The Fitness Odyssey

Fitness is not about reaching a specific milestone or achieving a certain look; it's about maintaining and improving your health throughout life. Whether you're just starting out on your fitness journey or have been at it for years, the practices outlined in this book are designed to help you stay active, healthy, and happy at every stage.

It's never too early - or too late - to begin. Even if you're just starting out, know that you're taking a crucial step toward a healthier future. Start small, build momentum, and celebrate every victory, no matter how small. If you're returning to fitness after a break, remember that every effort counts, and progress is possible at any age.

Setting Realistic Goals

At different stages of life, our goals and capabilities evolve. In your 20s and 30s, you might focus on building a strong foundation, trying new activities, and pushing your limits. In your 40s and 50s, the focus might shift to maintaining what you've built, preventing injury, and adapting to changes in energy levels and metabolism. In your 60s and beyond, the priority might be maintaining mobility, flexibility, and independence, with a focus on exercises that support everyday functionality.

The key is to set realistic, age-appropriate goals that challenge you without overwhelming you. Your fitness journey is personal, and it should evolve with you.

The Role of Mindset

Fitness isn't just physical - it's mental and emotional, too. As we explored in Chapter 16, *The Power of Habits,* and Chapter 15, *Motivation – Keeping the Fire Burning,* attitudes toward fitness often evolve with age, influenced by life experiences, shifting priorities, and physical capabilities. Cultivating a mindset that views fitness as a lifelong commitment is essential.

Staying motivated can be challenging, especially when faced with plateaus or life changes. It's important to set both short-term and long-term goals, celebrate small wins, and find joy in movement. Whether it's discovering a new form of exercise, revisiting an old favorite, or simply appreciating what your body can do, staying engaged is key to a sustainable fitness journey.

Life will inevitably bring changes - career shifts, family responsibilities, aging - and these can impact your fitness routine. The ability to adapt, embrace change, and continue prioritizing your health is crucial. Each stage of life offers new opportunities to reassess and refine your fitness approach, ensuring that it remains a source of joy and strength, rather than stress.

STAY FIT.. STAY FABULOUS !

Balancing Work, Life, Fitness

– Making Time for Wellness

The Modern-Day Juggle

Balancing the demands of a career, family, and personal life can often feel like juggling flaming swords while walking a tightrope. One of the biggest challenges people face on their fitness journey is finding time for health and wellness amid the chaos of everyday life. With modern work cultures increasingly demanding longer hours and constant availability, it's easy to push fitness and self-care to the bottom of your priority list.

Maintaining a balanced lifestyle is about harmonizing all aspects of your life, including work, family, fitness, and mental well-being. This chapter will provide you with practical strategies to integrate fitness seamlessly into your busy life, showing that you don't have to choose between success in your career and personal well-being.

(Refer to **Chapter 1: Why 40 is the New 30** to reinforce the importance of making fitness a priority in this stage of life and that age doesn't need to be a barrier.)

Section 1: The Myth of "Not Having Enough Time"

The most common reason people give for not exercising is "I don't have time." But in reality, it's not about having time - it's about making time. Often, the perception that there's no time for fitness comes from an all-or-nothing mindset - believing that a workout has to be an hour-long, intense session or it's not worth doing. The truth is, short bursts of activity can be just as effective when integrated into your routine, especially for busy schedules.

Practical Tips for Fitting Fitness into a Busy Schedule:

- **Micro Workouts**: As explained in **Chapter 7: The Power of Movement - Beyond the Gym**, short 10- to 15-minute workouts, such as bodyweight exercises or high-intensity interval training (HIIT), can be effective. Incorporating quick squats, push-ups, or planks during work breaks can help you maintain momentum.

- **Time Blocking for Fitness**: Schedule your workouts like any other important meeting. As mentioned in **Chapter 13: Creating a Personalized Fitness Plan**, fitness should be a part of your routine that fits into your life, not the other way around. Whether it's a 20-minute workout in the morning or a walk during lunch, planning it into your day makes it a non-negotiable priority.

- **Multitask Movement**: Incorporate more movement into your day as explained in **Chapter 7**. Take walking meetings, stand up and stretch while watching TV, or park further away to get more steps in. These little adjustments can add up over time.

Section 2: Setting Realistic Fitness Goals for Busy Lives

Setting realistic, achievable fitness goals that align with your workload and personal life is essential. Too often, people set ambitious goals that don't match their busy schedules, leading to frustration and burnout. **Chapter 13: Creating a Personalized Fitness Plan** highlights the importance of tailoring your fitness routine to your life, ensuring it's flexible enough to accommodate the ebbs and flows of daily responsibilities.

Practical Tips for Achievable Fitness Goals:

- **Weekly vs. Daily Goals**: As covered in **Chapter 16: The Power of Habits**, creating consistent habits is key. Aim for three to four workouts per week instead of daily, allowing flexibility during busy times. Weekly goals give you space to adjust your routine without feeling like you've failed.
- **Small, Measurable Changes**: Begin with small changes, as explained in **Chapter 16**. Whether it's walking 10,000 steps a day or committing to two 20-minute sessions a week, start with small, measurable goals that fit your schedule.
- **Tailor Your Routine**: Just like in **Chapter 13**, tailor your fitness plan to your preferences and time constraints. If you're a morning person, consider short, early workouts. If evenings are better, try a relaxing yoga session after work. Flexibility ensures long-term success.

Section 3: Fitness in the Office – Small Steps, Big Impact

For those working in sedentary office jobs, fitness can feel distant. However, there are many small ways to stay active, even during work hours. Sitting for extended periods not only leads to physical discomfort but also affects overall health, as discussed in **Chapter 7: The Power of Movement**.

Practical Tips for Office Fitness:

- **Standing Desks**: Using a standing desk, as mentioned in **Chapter 7**, can help reduce the harmful effects of sitting for prolonged periods. Standing or using an adjustable desk can improve posture and prevent the back pain associated with desk work.
- **Desk Exercises**: Incorporating desk exercises like stretches, leg raises, or shoulder rolls can prevent stiffness and improve circulation. In **Chapter 7**, we discussed how even small movements can count as NEAT (Non-Exercise Activity Thermogenesis) and contribute to staying fit.
- **Walking Meetings**: When possible, suggest walking meetings with colleagues. This not only helps you get moving but, as shown in **Chapter 7**, walking also improves creativity and focus.

Section 4: Healthy Eating When You're Always on the Go

When you're juggling a busy schedule, maintaining a healthy diet can be challenging. But making smart nutritional choices, even when you're pressed for time, is possible. **Part 3: Nutrition - Eating Smart, Not Less** introduced the concept of quantified nutrition and making conscious food choices, which ties directly into managing eating habits while busy.

Practical Tips for Healthy Eating on the Go:

- **Meal Prepping**: In **Chapter 9**, we talked about meal planning and preparing meals in advance. Even simple meal prep - like cooking chicken and vegetables for the week or portioning out healthy snacks - can keep you on track. Having ready-to-go meals prevents you from turning to fast food or unhealthy options.

- **Healthy Snacks**: Keep healthy snacks on hand, such as nuts, yogurt, or fruits. This helps curb hunger and keeps you from reaching for unhealthy snacks. Protein bars or roasted chickpeas are easy, portable, and nutrient-rich options.
- **Mindful Choices When Eating Out**: When dining out, refer back to **Chapter 11: Decoding Nutrition Labels**. Look for nutrient-dense foods, avoid hidden sugars and unhealthy fats, and request sauces or dressings on the side. This helps you make healthier choices without feeling deprived.

Section 5: Managing Stress and Mental Wellness

Work-related stress can derail both your mental and physical health, making it harder to stay on track with your fitness goals. **Chapter 14: Tracking Progress Without Losing Your Mind** highlighted the importance of mental wellness, and this section will emphasize how stress management is key to maintaining balance in your life.

Practical Tips for Managing Stress:

- **Mindfulness and Meditation**: In **Chapter 14**, we discussed how mindfulness practices like meditation can reduce stress and improve focus. Consider incorporating five to ten minutes of mindfulness meditation into your routine to reset during stressful periods.
- **The Role of Sleep**: As discussed extensively in **Chapter 4: Sleep - Your Secret Weapon**, sleep plays a crucial role in

managing stress and maintaining overall wellness. Poor sleep exacerbates stress, so ensuring adequate rest is fundamental.

- **Exercise as Stress Relief**: Physical activity can be one of the most effective ways to manage stress. Whether it's a quick walk or a workout session, as mentioned in **Chapter 7**, exercise helps release endorphins, which are natural stress relievers.

Conclusion: Striking the Right Balance

Achieving a balance between work, life, and fitness is an ongoing process. Just as discussed in **Chapter 13: Creating a Personalized Fitness Plan**, flexibility and consistency are key. The goal is to adapt your routine to fit your lifestyle, allowing it to evolve as your personal and professional life changes. Remember, there will be times when work takes priority and times when you can focus more on fitness, but by maintaining balance, you'll achieve long-term success.

Refer back to **Chapter 18: The Journey Continues** for encouragement to embrace fitness as a lifelong journey. The key takeaway? Fitness is not about perfection, but about finding what works for you - sustainably and flexibly.

Fad Diets, Fancy Foods, and the Science of Energy Balance

Introduction: Lost in the Noise of Nutrition

Picture this: You decide to lose weight and improve your health. You open social media and see conflicting advice everywhere.

- One influencer says, "Cut carbs completely. Keto is the way to lose fat!"
- Another swears by, "Skip breakfast - intermittent fasting is magic!"
- Your favorite wellness page shouts, "Buy organic, gluten-free quinoa and chia seeds!"

Suddenly, it feels like getting fit requires a Ph.D. in nutrition, a truckload of willpower, and a bank account big enough to buy exotic groceries every week. You're overwhelmed. You wonder:

"Is fitness only for people who can afford fancy foods and follow strict rules?"

The truth is far simpler. Nutrition isn't about trends, expensive ingredients, or magic fixes. It's about **understanding energy balance**, choosing foods that fit your life, and building habits you can sustain.

In this chapter, we'll explore two critical topics:

1. **The Illusion of Fad Diets:** Why they seem to work and why they fail in the long run.
2. **The Fancy Food Myth:** Why you don't need exotic superfoods for fitness.

By the end, you'll realize that achieving your fitness goals is simpler, cheaper, and far more achievable than you've been led to believe.

Part 1: The Illusion of Fad Diets

The Universal Truth Behind Every Diet

Every year, there's a new "revolutionary" diet claiming to be the **ultimate solution** for fat loss. Let's take a closer look at some of the most popular ones:

1. **The Ketogenic (Keto) Diet:** "Cut carbs to zero and eat fats to burn fat!"
2. **Intermittent Fasting:** "Skip meals to force your body into fat-burning mode."
3. **Juice Cleanses:** "Detoxify your body with liquid-only diets."
4. **Low-Fat Diets:** "Eliminate fats to reduce calories and lose weight."

Each of these diets comes wrapped in complicated "rules" and exciting claims. They sound scientific, but beneath the surface, there's only one reason they "work" for fat loss:

They create a calorie deficit.

We have discussed details about Calorie Balance in Chapter 2. Let's revisit what is Energy Balance and Calorie Deficit?

To understand weight loss, you must understand **energy balance** - a concept rooted in physics. Your body follows the basic principle of thermodynamics:

- **Calories In > Calories Out = Weight Gain**
- **Calories In < Calories Out = Weight Loss**
- **Calories In = Calories Out = Maintenance**

Calories are units of energy you get from food. Your body burns calories for everything - breathing, digesting food, moving, thinking, and even sleeping. If you consume fewer calories than your body needs, it taps into stored energy (body fat) to make up the deficit. This is **fat loss**.

Why Do Fad Diets "Work"?

Each fad diet creates a calorie deficit in disguise, but they package it in different ways:

1. **The Keto Diet:**

   o   You eliminate carbs, cutting out a major source of calories.
   o   Less variety in food = you eat fewer calories naturally.
   o   **Side Effect:** Water loss during the first few days gives the illusion of rapid weight loss.

2. **Intermittent Fasting (IF):**

   o   You skip meals, reducing your overall calorie intake.
   o   Eating for only 6-8 hours naturally limits how much you can eat.

3. **Juice Cleanses and Detox Diets:**

   o   Liquid-only diets drastically reduce calorie intake.
   o   While you lose weight quickly, it's mostly water and muscle - not sustainable fat loss.

4. **Low-Fat Diets:**

   o   Removing fats reduces overall calorie intake (since fats are calorie-dense).

Key Point: These diets work *not* because of their rules or "magic" but because they help you eat fewer calories than you burn.

The Problems with Fad Diets

While fad diets may work in the short term, they create bigger problems over time:

1. **They're Unsustainable:**

   - Can you cut carbs forever? Can you drink only juice for weeks?
   - The minute you return to "normal" eating, the weight comes back.

2. **They Lead to Nutritional Imbalances:**

   - Keto diets lack fiber and certain vitamins.
   - Low-fat diets deprive you of essential fatty acids and fat-soluble vitamins.

3. **They Cause the Yo-Yo Effect:**

   - Rapid weight loss often leads to rapid weight regain. You lose motivation, and the cycle continues.

Analogy:

"Fad diets are like crash courses - you cram for results, but forget everything as soon as the test ends. Sustainable habits, on the other hand, are like lifelong education."

What's the Alternative?

Instead of hopping from one extreme diet to another, focus on:

1. **A Moderate Calorie Deficit:** Aim for a 10-20% reduction in calories from your maintenance intake.
2. **Balanced Nutrition:** Include all macronutrients - proteins, carbs, and fats.
3. **Flexibility:** Enjoy foods you love in moderation.

Remember: The best diet is not the "trendiest" one; it's the one you can follow for life.

Part 2: Nutrition Doesn't Require Fancy Foods

Busting the Fancy Food Myth

Have you ever felt that fitness is out of reach because you can't afford expensive groceries like quinoa, avocados, almond milk, and chia seeds?

Here's the reality: **Your body doesn't care whether calories and nutrients come from a ₹500 bag of quinoa or a simple bowl of rice.**

Superfoods vs. Local Foods: A Practical Comparison

Let's compare "fancy" foods with their local, affordable alternatives:

Fancy Food	Local Food	Why Local Foods Work
Quinoa	Rice or Roti	Both provide carbs for energy.
Chia Seeds	Flaxseeds or Sesame Seeds	Both are rich in omega-3s and fiber.
Almond Milk	Regular Milk or Curd	Curd has more protein and probiotics.
Avocado	Ghee or Groundnuts	Both offer healthy fats when eaten moderately.

Example:

"Think of dal-rice with ghee and vegetables. It's a complete meal - balanced, nutritious, and far cheaper than an avocado toast with almond milk coffee."

Why Local Foods Are Better

1. **Affordable:** No need to spend thousands on imported groceries.
2. **Easily Available:** Traditional foods are part of our culture and diet.
3. **Nutritionally Adequate:** A home-cooked meal provides all essential nutrients.

Key Message: Fitness isn't about eating "Instagrammable" meals. It's about choosing nutrient-dense foods that fit your budget and lifestyle.

Simplifying Your Nutrition

Here's how you can keep it simple:

1. **Eat Whole, Local Foods:** Dal, rice, roti, vegetables, eggs, paneer, and fruits are enough.
2. **Focus on Balance:** Include protein, carbs, and fats in every meal.
3. **Ignore Trends:** You don't need "superfoods." You need consistency.

Conclusion: Keep It Simple, Sustainable, and Effective

Nutrition doesn't need to be complicated, expensive, or trendy. At the end of the day:

1. **Fad Diets fail** because they're unsustainable.
2. **Fancy Foods are optional** - local, simple foods are just as effective.

Focus on what works:

- **Energy Balance:** Calories in vs. calories out.

- **Simple Foods:** Eat foods you love and can afford.
- **Sustainability:** Build habits you can follow for life.

Fitness is not a privilege for the wealthy or the disciplined. It's a result of small, consistent steps that anyone can take.

Take the pressure off yourself, stick to the basics, and trust the process.

Health After 40 - Fitness and Nutrition as Preventive Tools

Introduction: Understanding Health After 40

> *Before diving in, it's crucial to note that this chapter offers general guidance, not medical advice. For specific health concerns, always consult healthcare professionals. The strategies in this chapter are meant to complement medical treatment, not replace it.*

As we age, our bodies undergo changes that can affect overall health. After 40, medical conditions like heart disease, diabetes, hypertension, osteoporosis, and hormonal imbalances become more common. However, many of these conditions can be managed or even prevented through lifestyle choices centered on fitness, nutrition, and wellness.

(*Refer to* **Chapter 1: Why 40 is the New 30** *for more on embracing this age as a phase of growth, where health should become a priority.*)

Section 1: Common Health Issues for Men and Women After 40

Here, we explore the common health challenges faced by men and women as they age. While some issues are gender-specific, many affect both.

A. Women's Health Concerns After 40

Menopause and Hormonal Imbalances: Hormonal fluctuations during menopause can cause symptoms like hot flashes, mood swings, and decreased bone density.

Link to Fitness/Nutrition: Resistance training (see **Chapter 3: Why Strength Training is Non-Negotiable After 40**) helps maintain bone density, while a diet rich in calcium, vitamin D, and phytoestrogens (like flaxseeds and soy) supports hormonal balance.

Bone Health: With reduced estrogen levels, the risk of osteoporosis increases.

Link to Fitness/Nutrition: As noted in **Part 3**, weight-bearing exercises and nutrient-dense diets that include calcium and vitamin D are critical for maintaining bone health.

Thyroid Issues: Hypothyroidism is more common in women over 40, leading to symptoms like weight gain and fatigue.

Link to Fitness/Nutrition: A balanced diet with iodine-rich foods (e.g., seaweed, fish) and regular physical activity (explained in **Chapter 7: The Power of Movement - Beyond the Gym**) can help manage thyroid health.

Breast Health: Breast cancer risk increases with age.

Link to Fitness/Nutrition: Regular exercise (see **Chapter 7**) and a diet rich in fruits, vegetables, and lean protein (covered in **Part 3: Nutrition - Eating Smart, Not Less**) can support breast health.

B. Men's Health Concerns After 40

Cardiovascular Health: Risk factors for heart disease like high blood pressure and cholesterol increase after 40.

Link to Fitness/Nutrition: Cardiovascular exercises (**Chapter 7**) and heart-healthy diets (**Chapter 8**) that focus on reducing saturated fats and increasing fiber can help manage these risks.

Testosterone Decline: Reduced testosterone levels can lead to muscle loss, increased body fat, and decreased energy.

Link to Fitness/Nutrition: Strength training (**Chapter 3**) and a diet with healthy fats, zinc, and vitamin D (discussed in **Chapter 8**) can help maintain muscle mass and energy levels.

Prostate Health: Risk of prostate enlargement and cancer increases after 40.

Link to Fitness/Nutrition: Foods like tomatoes, green tea, and cruciferous vegetables support prostate health, as outlined in **Chapter 8**.

C. Health Concerns for Both Genders

Metabolic Slowdown: Metabolism slows down with age, making weight management more challenging.

Link to Fitness/Nutrition: Incorporating strength training (**Chapter 3**) and cardio (**Chapter 7**), along with a protein-rich diet (**Chapter 8**), can boost metabolism and maintain muscle mass.

Joint Health: Joint pain and stiffness can increase due to arthritis or prolonged inactivity.

Link to Fitness/Nutrition: Low-impact exercises like swimming or yoga (**Chapter 7**) help maintain joint flexibility, while foods rich in omega-3s (e.g., fatty fish, walnuts) reduce inflammation (**Chapter 10**).

Mental Health: Anxiety, depression, and cognitive decline may become more prominent due to stress and hormonal changes.

Link to Fitness/Nutrition: Regular exercise (**Chapter 7**), especially cardio, and diets rich in omega-3s and B vitamins (**Chapter 8**), can support mental well-being.

Diabetes and Blood Sugar Management: Risk of type 2 diabetes increases with age, especially with other risk factors like obesity or a sedentary lifestyle.

Link to Fitness/Nutrition: A balanced diet with controlled carbohydrate intake (**Chapter 8**) and regular exercise (**Chapter 7**) are crucial for managing or preventing type 2 diabetes.

Section 2: How Fitness and Nutrition Can Help

This section links the health challenges discussed above to the core principles of fitness and nutrition described in the book.

A. Strength Training and Bone Health

As explained in Chapter 3, strength training not only preserves muscle mass but also plays a crucial role in maintaining bone density, preventing age-related bone loss, and improving overall strength and balance.

Practical Tip: Incorporate 2-3 days of strength training into your routine, focusing on major muscle groups.

B. Cardio for Heart Health and Metabolism

Chapter 7 emphasizes the role of cardiovascular exercises in improving heart health, boosting metabolism, and managing weight. Cardio workouts can help control blood pressure, reduce cholesterol, and enhance lung capacity.

Practical Tip: Aim for at least 150 minutes of moderate-intensity cardio per week, spread across various activities you enjoy, such as brisk walking, cycling, or swimming.

C. Nutrient-Dense Diets for Hormonal Balance and Weight Management

Chapter 8 covers the importance of a nutrient-dense diet in regulating hormones, managing weight, and supporting metabolic health. The right balance of macronutrients and micronutrients can help mitigate hormonal imbalances and slow down metabolic decline.

Practical Tip: Include lean proteins, healthy fats, whole grains, and plenty of vegetables in your diet, while limiting sugar and processed foods.

D. Sleep and Stress Management

As detailed in **Chapter 4**, adequate sleep and stress management are key to maintaining hormonal balance, cognitive function, and overall well-being. Poor sleep and high stress levels can exacerbate many age-related health issues.

Practical Tip: Prioritize 7-9 hours of quality sleep each night and incorporate stress-relief techniques like meditation or deep breathing.

Section 3: Empowering Health with Preventive Lifestyle Changes

While fitness and nutrition are powerful tools for managing health after 40, adopting a proactive approach to regular medical screenings and preventive measures is crucial.

A. Regular Health Check-Ups

Routine medical screenings for blood pressure, cholesterol, blood sugar, and cancer are essential for early detection and prevention of age-related conditions.

Practical Tip: Schedule annual health check-ups, including gender-specific screenings (e.g., mammograms, prostate exams). These screenings, coupled with a consistent fitness and nutrition plan from **Chapter 13: Creating a Personalized Fitness Plan**, allow for a well-rounded approach to health management.

B. Incorporating Fitness and Nutrition as Preventive Medicine

As detailed throughout the book, consistent exercise, a balanced diet, and adequate sleep serve as powerful preventive measures against many chronic diseases.

Practical Tip: Follow the strategies outlined in earlier chapters on meal planning (**Chapter 9**), personalized fitness (**Chapter 13**), and sleep optimization (**Chapter 4**) to develop a lifestyle that supports long-term health.

C. Emphasizing a Holistic Approach

The integration of fitness, nutrition, mental well-being, and regular medical consultations forms a holistic approach to health after 40.

Practical Tip: Make time for mental wellness activities like meditation (**Chapter 14: Tracking Progress Without Losing Your Mind**) and ensure regular communication with healthcare professionals to align your fitness regimen with any medical needs.

Conclusion: The Role of Fitness and Nutrition in Aging Well

This chapter has emphasized that while aging brings specific health risks, a proactive approach centered around fitness, nutrition, and regular medical care can significantly reduce these risks. The strategies and insights from earlier chapters provide a framework for maintaining physical and mental well-being well into your 40s, 50s, and beyond. Remember, the advice in this book is meant to be a guide, not a substitute for professional medical care. Always consult with healthcare providers for personalized guidance.

Companion Website - Fitness & Nutrition Tools/Guides

Explore a Growing Library of Fitness & Nutrition Resources:

To make your journey easier and more effective, I've compiled a collection of **downloadable tools and guides** that you can **access anytime**. These resources are designed to help you stay organized, track progress, and make fitness a sustainable part of your lifestyle.

Here's what you'll find on the site:

- **Fitness Progress Trackers:** Stay motivated by logging your workouts, tracking improvements, and setting clear goals. Whether you're aiming to build strength, lose fat, or improve endurance, these trackers will help you **visualize your progress** and keep you accountable.
- **Meal Planning Templates:** Simplify your nutrition with structured meal planning sheets. These templates help you **plan balanced meals** for the week, ensure adequate macronutrient intake, and save time in the kitchen by organizing grocery lists and meal prep.
- **Workout Routines:** Whether you're a beginner or experienced, you'll find a variety of workout plans tailored to different fitness levels and goals. These routines are easy to follow and provide structured training plans that keep you **on track and progressing**.
- **Gym Workout Guides:** Confused about gym workouts? These guides break down different types of exercises, proper form, and how to structure your gym sessions for maximum results. From **strength training splits** to **full-**

body workouts, these guides will help you **train effectively and confidently**.

- **Replacement Ingredients Guide:** Want to tweak your meals but unsure what to substitute? This handy guide provides **macronutrient breakdowns and substitution options** for common household ingredients, allowing you to **customize meals without compromising nutrition**.

More to Come!

This is **just the beginning**! Over time, I'll be adding **more tools, guides, and resources** to help you stay consistent, improve your knowledge, and make lasting progress.

📌 Access the resources here:

🌐 https://agelessfitness40.wordpress.com/

You'll also find a **growing community** where fitness enthusiasts can share experiences, discuss challenges, and stay motivated. **Your fitness journey is personal, but you're never alone - let's grow stronger together!**

Fitness and Nutrition-Educational Resources

1. **The American Council on Exercise (ACE)**
   https://www.acefitness.org/

   o   Focuses on fitness education, offering certifications, workout programs, and health information.

2. **American Heart Association – Healthy Eating https://www.heart.org/en/healthy-living/healthy-eating**

   o   Focuses on heart-healthy eating tips, recipes, and guidelines for a balanced diet.

3. **Bodybuilding.com**
   https://www.bodybuilding.com/

   o   Offers a vast library of workout routines, nutrition tips, and supplements for fitness enthusiasts.

4. **Centers for Disease Control and Prevention (CDC) – Nutrition**
   https://www.cdc.gov/nutrition/

   o   Offers resources on healthy eating, weight management, and physical activity.

5. **Eatright.org**
   https://www.eatright.org/

   o   The Academy of Nutrition and Dietetics' site offering articles on diet, nutrition, and health.

6. **Examine.com**
   https://examine.com/

   o   Offers unbiased research summaries on supplements and nutrition, focusing on evidence-based findings.

7. **Fittr**
   https://www.fittr.com/

   - A comprehensive platform offering fitness and nutrition advice, personalized coaching, and community support.

8. **Greatist**
   https://greatist.com/

   - A wellness site offering advice on fitness, health, mental well-being, and healthy eating.

9. **Harvard T.H. Chan School of Public Health – The Nutrition Source**
   https://www.hsph.harvard.edu/nutritionsource/

   - Offers evidence-based guidance on healthy eating, nutrition news, and research findings.

10. **Healthline – Nutrition**
    https://www.healthline.com/nutrition

    - Covers a wide range of nutrition topics, including diet plans, food analysis, and wellness tips.

11. **Livestrong – Fitness**
    https://www.livestrong.com/cat/fitness

    - A resource for fitness routines, healthy living tips, and nutrition advice.

12. **Mayo Clinic – Fitness and Nutrition**
    https://www.mayoclinic.org/healthy-lifestyle/fitness

    - Provides expert advice on fitness routines, nutrition, and overall health.

13. **MyFitnessPal**
    https://www.myfitnesspal.com/

    o   A popular app and website for tracking diet and exercise, offering a community and tools for weight loss.

14. **National Institutes of Health (NIH) – Nutrition**
    https://www.nutrition.gov/

    o   A comprehensive resource on nutrition, including dietary guidelines, food sources, and more.

15. **Precision Nutrition**
    https://www.precisionnutrition.com/

    o   Provides personalized nutrition coaching, articles, and tips on healthy eating and fitness.

16. **Self – Fitness**
    https://www.self.com/fitness

    o   Provides workout plans, fitness tips, and articles on staying active and healthy.

17. **Shape – Nutrition**
    https://www.shape.com/healthy-eating/diet-tips

    o   Provides recipes, healthy eating tips, and advice on maintaining a balanced diet.

18. **Verywell Fit**
    https://www.verywellfit.com/

    o   Offers comprehensive articles on fitness, nutrition, and wellness, backed by experts.

19. **WebMD – Diet & Weight Management**
    https://www.webmd.com/diet/default.htm

    o   Offers practical advice on diet, nutrition, and managing a healthy weight.

20. **World Health Organization (WHO) – Nutrition and Physical Activity**
    https://www.who.int/health-topics/nutrition

    o   Provides global guidelines on nutrition and physical activity for maintaining health.

REFERENCES

American Heart Association. (2024). *Updated Guidelines on Cardiovascular Health.* Reference - https://www.heart.org

Centers for Disease Control and Prevention (CDC). (2024). *Latest Insights on Bone Health and Aging.* Reference - https://www.cdc.gov

Harvard T.H. Chan School of Public Health. (2024). *The Nutrition Source: Understanding Macronutrients.* Reference - https://www.hsph.harvard.edu/nutritionsource

Mayo Clinic. (2024). *Perimenopause and Menopause: Managing Symptoms Naturally.* Reference - https://www.mayoclinic.org

National Institutes of Health (NIH). (2024). *Exercise Guidelines for Adults Over 40.* Reference - https://www.nih.gov

World Health Organization (WHO). (2024). *Global Physical Activity Guidelines: An Update.* Reference - https://www.who.int

U.S. Department of Agriculture (USDA). (2024). *Decoding Nutrition Labels for Healthier Choices.* Reference - https://www.usda.gov

National Osteoporosis Foundation. (2024). *Strategies for Preventing Osteoporosis.* Reference - https://www.nof.org

WebMD. (2024). *Menopause: Lifestyle Changes, Therapies, and Health Tips.* Reference - https://www.webmd.com

Harvard Medical School. (2024). *The Impact of Sleep on Long-Term Health.* Reference - https://www.health.harvard.edu

National Institute of Nutrition, India. (2024). *Dietary Guidelines for Indians - A Manual.* Reference - https://www.nin.res.in

References

Indian Council of Medical Research (ICMR). (2024). *Nutritional Requirements and Recommended Dietary Allowances for Indians.* Reference - https://www.icmr.gov.in

Ministry of Health and Family Welfare, Government of India. (2024). *Guidelines for Physical Activity in India.* Reference - https://www.mohfw.gov.in

National Institute of Mental Health and Neurosciences (NIMHANS), India. (2024). *Mental Health and Stress Management: A Guide for Indians.* Reference - https://nimhans.ac.in

Public Health Foundation of India (PHFI). (2024). *Heart Health in India: Emerging Trends and Preventative Measures.* Reference - https://phfi.org

All India Institute of Medical Sciences (AIIMS). (2024). *Menopause Management: Indian Perspectives.* Reference - https://www.aiims.edu

Cleveland Clinic. (2024). *Understanding Bone Health: Latest Research and Recommendations.* Reference - https://my.clevelandclinic.org

The Lancet. (2024). *Impact of Diet on Cardiovascular Health: A Global Perspective.* Reference - https://www.thelancet.com

Journal of Clinical Endocrinology & Metabolism. (2024). *Hormone Therapy and Long-Term Health in Women.* Reference - https://academic.oup.com/jcem

Jitendra Chouksey. (2024). *Lose Fat, Get Fittr.* Reference - https://www.amazon.in/LOSE-FAT-GET-FITTR-SCIENCE

Jitendra Chouksey. (2024). Get Shredded. Reference - **https://d26awh6k8vkquc.cloudfront.net/fittr/GetShredded_V4.pdf**

www.ingramcontent.com/pod-product-compliance
Lightning Source LLC
Chambersburg PA
CBHW031023160726
47991CB00005B/1849